SECOND EDITION

# Evidence-Based Falls Prevention

## A STUDY GUIDE FOR NURSES

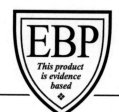

EBP
*This product
is evidence
based*

**Carole Eldridge, DNP, RN, CNAA-BC**

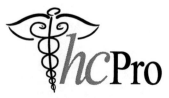

*Evidence-Based Falls Prevention: A Study Guide for Nurses, Second Edition* is published by HCPro, Inc.

HCPro, Inc., provides information resources for the healthcare industry.

HCPro, Inc., is not affiliated in any way with The Joint Commission, which owns the JCAHO and Joint Commission trademarks.

Carole Eldridge, DNP, RN, CNAA-BC, Author
Elaine Graf, PhD, RN, PNP, Reviewer
Rebecca Hendren, Managing Editor
Lindsey Cardarelli, Associate Editor
Emily Sheahan, Group Publisher
Shane Katz, Cover Designer
Jackie Diehl Singer, Graphic Artist

Paul Singer, Layout Artist
Audrey Doyle, Copyeditor
Sada Preisch, Proofreader
Darren Kelly, Books Production Supervisor
Susan Darbyshire, Art Director
Claire Cloutier, Production Manager
Jean St. Pierre, Director of Operations

Advice given is general. Readers should consult professional counsel for specific legal, ethical, or clinical questions.

"Magnet Recognition Program®" is a registered trademark of the American Nurses Credentialing Center (ANCC). HCPro, Inc., and The Greeley Company's products and services are not a part of, nor endorsed by, the ANCC.

Arrangements can be made for quantity discounts. For more information, contact:

HCPro, Inc.
P.O. Box 1168
Marblehead, MA 01945
Telephone: 800/650-6787 or 781/639-1872
Fax: 781/639-2982
E-mail: *customerservice@hcpro.com*

**Visit HCPro at its World Wide Web sites: *www.hcpro.com* and *www.hcmarketplace.com***

# Contents

# Contents

# Figures

## Carole Eldridge, DNP, RN, CNAA-BC

**Carole Eldridge, DNP, RN, CNAA-BC,** is a board-certified nurse administrator, advanced, with extensive experience in starting and managing healthcare companies. Eldridge has opened and operated several Medicare and private-duty home health agencies, a hospice, a medical equipment company, and a healthcare publishing company, overseeing a four-state home care company as chief executive officer for several years. She has served as both national staff development coordinator and vice president of resident and quality services for a large assisted-living company. Eldridge has written and published more than 60 training publications for unlicensed attendants in long-term care as well as a number of articles for professional journals. Currently working as an assistant professor in a university's college of nursing, Eldridge speaks often to industry and community groups on staff development and training, employee retention, career ladder programs, and healthcare administration. She is a partner in CareTrack Resources, Inc., a firm that provides continuing education for administrators and nurses and consulting services for healthcare companies.

## ELAINE GRAF, PHD, RN, PNP

**Elaine Graf, PhD, RN, PNP** has been a pediatric nurse for her entire professional career. In her position as Research and Funding Coordinator at Children's Memorial Medical Center in Chicago, she supports and encourages professional development and research endeavors of the nursing staff. As ANCC® Magnet Recognition Program director, she has overseen a successful initial designation in 2001 and redesignation in 2005. Dr. Graf has been instrumental in establishing internal funding programs that support over $100,000 per year in research and special project initiatives. Her area of research focus is the prevention of inpatient pediatric falls. This research has resulted in a validated predictor model, *The General Risk Assessment for Pediatric In-patient Falls Scale (GRAF PIF)*, which is being used in over 130 pediatric facilities. Dr. Graf has multiple publications and has presented papers at numerous national and international conferences. She is a member of Sigma Theta Tau, The Society of Pediatric Nurses, The American Nurses Association, and The Illinois Council on Nurse Resources.

## BENEFITS OF EVIDENCE-BASED FALLS PREVENTION, SECOND EDITION

*Evidence-Based Falls Prevention, Second Edition*, is a complete guide that will help you discover the risk factor assessment and prevention strategies your facility needs to implement a successful falls prevention policy. With an effective falls prevention program in place, your nurses can keep patients safe and exceed compliance requirements.

Versions of the guide's tools and templates can be found on the accompanying CD-ROM. Put your organization's name on the forms, customize them to fit your needs, and print them out for immediate staff use.

## HOW TO USE THE FILES ON YOUR CD-ROM

To adapt any of the files to your own facility, simply follow the instructions below to open the CD-ROM.

If you have trouble reading the forms, click on "View," and then "Normal." To adapt the forms, save them first to your own hard drive or disk (by clicking "File," then "Save as," and changing the system to your own). Then change the information to fit your facility, and add or delete any items that you wish to change.

The following file names correspond with tools listed in the manual:

| File name | Document |
| --- | --- |
| Figure 2.1 | Functional assessment tool |
| Figure 2.2 | Problem list |
| Figure 2.3 | Interdisciplinary plan of care tool sample |
| Figure 2.4 | Interdisciplinary team conference assessment |
| Figure 3.1 | Nonmodifiable intrinsic fall risk factors |

**Evidence-Based Falls Prevention, Second Edition**

| File name | Document |
|-----------|----------|
| Figure 3.2 | Medical conditions that increase fall risk |
| Figure 3.3 | Cardiovascular causes of falls |
| Figure 4.1 | Effective exercise programs tested in randomized controlled trials |
| Figure 4.2 | Daily staff considerations for fall prevention |
| Figure 4.3 | Frequent causes of OH |
| Figure 4.4 | Nonpharmacological treatments for OH |
| Figure 5.1 | Fall assessment guidelines |
| Figure 5.2 | Sample Morse risk assessment tool |
| Figure 5.3 | Fall risk evaluation tool |
| Figure 5.4 | Post-fall assessment/response decision tree |
| Figure 5.5 | Fall documentation and root-cause analysis |
| Figure 5.6 | Hazard identification documentation |
| Figure 5.7 | Fall-tracking document |
| Figure 5.8 | Falls standard audit |
| Figure 6.1 | Head-injury monitoring plan |
| Figure 6.2 | Initial note documentation |
| Figure 6.3 | Nursing documentation for falls |
| Figure 7.1 | CHAMPS pediatric fall risk assessment tool |

## Installation instructions

This product was designed for the Windows operating system and includes Word files that will run under Windows 95/98 or greater. The CD-ROM will work on all PCs and most Macintosh systems. To run the files, take the following steps:

1. Insert the CD into your CD-ROM drive.
2. Double-click on the "My Computer" icon, next double-click on the CD drive icon.
3. Double-click on the files you wish to open.
4. Adapt the files by moving the cursor over the areas you wish to change, highlighting them, and typing in the new information using Microsoft Word.
5. To save a file to your facility's system, click on "File" and then click on "Save As." Select the location where you wish to save the file and then click on "Save."
6. To print a document, click on "File" and then click on "Print."

# CHAPTER 1:

# Introduction

# Introduction

## The problem

Falls are the single most significant adverse event experienced in hospitals, negatively affecting physical and emotional health, as well as overall quality of life.[1] Falls are a critical problem in all healthcare organizations, accounting for a significant number of injuries due to inadequate caregiver communication; incomplete assessment, reassessment, and training of new staff; inadequate staffing levels; malfunction or misuse of equipment; and insufficient education of the patient and his or her family.

The data are alarming: Falls are the largest single category of reported incidents in hospitals. Patient falls are often cited as the second most frequent cause of harm for patients, topped only by medication errors. Falls are the leading cause of nonfatal injuries and trauma-related hospitalizations in the United States. Two percent to 4% of all patients fall, and 2% to 6% of these falls result in a serious injury, such as a fracture. In the United States, one out of every three people aged 65 and older falls each year.[2] Falls are a leading cause of traumatic brain injuries and morbidity, affect all patient populations, and occur regularly among patients in acute care facilities.

According to the Centers for Disease Control and Prevention (CDC), U.S. medical costs for fall-related injuries equal $20.2 billion and are expected to rise to $32.4 billion by 2020. The latest CDC report, issued in 2006, notes that in 2003, more than 13,700 people age 65 or older died of fall-related injuries, and another 1.8 million were treated in emergency departments for nonfatal injuries related to falls. The financial repercussions and adverse consequences (including fracture, head injury, depression, and fear of falling) associated with patient falls are among the most serious risk management issues that hospitals face. Additionally, on average, an elderly patient who falls will stay 18 days longer than originally planned.[3]

Because of the potential adverse consequences associated with patient falls, each hospital must create a comprehensive program to reduce falls. There is no single fall-prevention program that works for all patients in every healthcare setting. A successful multifaceted program analyzes how and where falls happen, targets the unit where falls are most frequent, varies program elements to fit patients' needs, ensures that reporting the circumstances of patient falls is nonpunitive, assesses every patient for fall risk, and reeducates staff periodically. In addition to a comprehensive fall-prevention program, a predictive, multidisciplinary assessment of fall risk of patients at admission, including their history of falls, depression, dizziness or vertigo, confusion or dementia, and cognitive impairment, is essential to the delivery of optimal patient care.

Additionally, as one of its 2008 National Patient Safety Goals, The Joint Commission (formerly JCAHO) requires that hospitals reduce the risk of patient harm as a result of falls and will look for documentation pertaining to this requirement. The goal also states that hospitals must implement a fall reduction program that includes an evaluation of the program's effectiveness.

And recently, under the new payment policy of the Centers for Medicare and Medicaid Services (CMS), hospitals will cease to be compensated for the treatment of "reasonably preventable" conditions required during patient stays, including injuries from patient falls. This rule was mandated by a 2005 law and takes effect in October 2008, emphasizing the critical need for hospitals to focus on falls-prevention strategies.

## The costs and risks

Across many industries, plaintiffs' attorneys and insurance companies examine several factors when considering the potential for liability. Businesses that are susceptible to lawsuits and insurance claims typically have the following characteristics in common:

1. They provide services that are potentially dangerous and could cause harmful mistakes.
2. They are subject to intense scrutiny by state and federal regulatory agencies, the public, and the media.
3. They feature complex, interdependent systems supported by multiple processes and disciplines.

Acutecare facilities feature each of these characteristics. Plaintiffs' attorneys can view hospitals as a source of potentially significant financial compensation, and insurance carriers can see the industry as a source of significant potential losses.

# The goals

In order to optimize patient care, The Joint Commission included falls prevention as one of its patient safety goals approved for 2008. The 2008 National Patient Safety Goals apply to the nearly 16,000 accredited healthcare organizations and programs, including ambulatory care and surgery centers, office-based surgery sites, assisted-living facilities, behavioral healthcare settings, home healthcare environments, nursing homes, laboratories, and hospitals. The Joint Commission first introduced its National Patient Safety Goals in an effort to improve patient safety. Each goal contains a set of evidence-based, specific requirements that identify opportunities for reducing risk to patients by pinpointing potential problems in critical aspects of care. Each year, The Joint Commission solicits feedback from healthcare professionals who review the current National Patient Safety Goals and make recommendations based on each goal's relevance, priority, clarity, ability to measure compliance, time needed to implement, and cost of implementation.

A patient falls goal that required healthcare organizations to reduce the risk of patient harm resulting from falls was first introduced in 2005, but the goal was revised in 2006 to include requirements for fall-reduction programs. Now, in 2008, The Joint Commission will be looking for evidence of well-developed and evaluated fall prevention programs. Organizations will be required to articulate a clear fall prevention program, discuss fall and injury rates, and show clear evidence of review of fall prevention interventions and changes made to further enhance fall prevention. All accredited organizations are surveyed for implementation of the goals and requirements. Surveyors look for evidence of implementation, review relevant documentation, and question leadership about how consistently the organization implements action into a care plan and what level of monitoring occurs after it implements each goal.

The falls prevention goal included in The Joint Commission's 2008 National Patient Safety Goals reads as follows:

> **Goal: Reduce the risk of patient harm resulting from falls.**
> - Implement a fall reduction program including an evaluation of the effectiveness of the program.

## The solution

There is no one-size-fits-all solution to the problem of falling. There is, however, a single main goal that every healthcare provider should work toward: prevention. Although it may not be possible to prevent every fall, most falls are preventable. Each fall prevented is one less potential injury, fracture, head trauma, or death. The goal of this book is to help healthcare providers learn how to prevent as many falls as possible, thereby preserving the mobility, qualify of life, and independence of patients.

## References

1. Wilson, E.B. (1998). "Preventing patient falls." AACN *Clinical Issues* 9: 100–108.

2. National Center for Injury Prevention and Control.

3. Swift, C.G. (2001). "Care of older people: Falls late in life and their consequences: Implementing effective services." *British Medical Journal* 322: 855–858.

# CHAPTER 2:

# Planning care through screening and assessment

# Planning care through screening and assessment

## Learning objectives

After reading this chapter, the participant should be able to:

- State a goal for performing an assessment
- Explain why documentation is important
- Describe the two phases of nursing assessment
- Identify elements of the functional screen

## Overview of the screening and assessment process and the multidisciplinary approach to planning care

An assessment of a patient's fall risk is critical to delivering the best nursing care. The goal of performing a screening assessment and developing a plan of care is to improve outcomes for the patient. What the clinician does or does not notice, teach, act on, report, or intervene upon greatly affects patient outcomes. The clinician determines what kind of care is required to meet the patient's needs by conducting an appropriate assessment. When the screening is complete and the assessment is thorough, the clinician is able to provide more effective and efficient care.

At admission, all patients receive a complete assessment that includes their physical, psychological, and social status. The scope and intensity of the initial screening assessment can be broadened based upon the patient's diagnosis, care setting, response to care, and previous treatments. It is during this initial screening assessment that the patient-identified needs begin to evolve. This evolution is the first step in the development of a plan of care. Caregivers develop criteria to be used as a guide for placing patients in a specific care setting or providing them with appropriate assistance during their inpatient stay.

Assessment involves the collection of data relevant to the patient's health status. Data are classified into two categories: subjective and objective. Subjective data can be obtained from the patient directly or indirectly (that is, they can be observed), but they cannot be measured. Objective data are observable and measurable.

Surveyors assess how staff members work together toward the benefit of patients. Each discipline should provide the patient with the best possible treatment plan. Up-to-date, objective patient information is essential in order for staff members to make the most appropriate recommendations.

Sharing patient information improves the probability that other healthcare professionals involved in the patient's care can achieve successful interventions and outcomes. Only through a cooperative team approach can we ensure that the best outcomes are achieved for the patients we treat. Lack of objective data can compromise and potentially threaten the health of the very people we serve. A mechanism should exist to ensure that assessment data are available to all appropriate healthcare providers.

Documentation demonstrates the staff's compliance with the standards for assessment and care of patients. Documentation should be accurate, brief, complete, objective, comprehensive, and legible. It must show that the staff thoroughly assessed the patient's condition, clearly identified the problems being treated, created a care plan that specifically addressed those problems, and continually evaluated the patient's status. The Joint Commission surveyors will assess compliance through observing, interviewing clinicians, and reviewing documentation.

Use a multidisciplinary patient assessment admission form to provide complete and concise documentation of the patient's initial assessment. Based on the initial screening assessment, which is generally performed by the nursing staff, all patients receive an initial clinical assessment performed by disciplines appropriate to their needs. For example, if an initial screening assessment identifies that a patient is at nutritional risk, the nutrition staff would be consulted, and a full assessment by a registered dietitian would follow. The clinical assessment provides the clinical team with information to develop a patient-specific plan of care, which identifies the patient's problem and needs. The initial patient assessment occurs at the time of admission and is usually within the patient's primary care setting. All patients are systematically and continuously assessed.

# PC.2.120

The hospital defines in writing the time frame(s) for conducting the initial assessment(s).

The Joint Commission allows the organization to establish its own internal time frame for completion of assessments except for the assessments that are specified in PC.2.120. For cases where a patient has been identified through the "screening assessment" to need a more extensive assessment of a specific system by a professional in that discipline, the organization's policy establishes a time frame for the secondary assessment. The initial screening assessment is generally completed within the first day of admission. When the organization defines the time frame for the secondary assessment, it needs to consider the type of patient, complexity of the patient's illness, length of time the patient will require care, and any other factors that impact the patient's care.

The organization's assessment policy must include the data gathered by the different clinical disciplines when completing a patient assessment and the time frame under which they are expected to complete their assessments:

- History and physical must be completed within 24 hours (this information must not be older than 30 days and must be updated at the time of admission)
- Nursing assessment must be completed within 24 hours
- Nutritional screening must be completed within 24 hours
- Functional screening must be completed within 24 hours

The organization's patient assessment admission form contains data that are used to assess the patient by the different disciplines and the date and time of the assessment.

The surveyor will conduct a record review and might inspect the organization's policy on patient assessment. Some questions a surveyor could ask during an interview with the staff include the following:

- Is there an established time frame in which your discipline must complete a patient assessment?
- Do you always complete the assessment within this established time frame?

You will comply with PC.2.120 by simply defining the time frames for specified settings and services and by holding the staff accountable for meeting them.

## Nursing assessment

The nurse focuses primarily on providing continuity of care for the patient. In the nursing process, the nurse collaborates with the patient to meet his or her needs. Remember one of the first lessons nurses are taught in nursing school: assess, plan, implement, and evaluate. For a nurse to prepare an individualized formal plan of care for the patient, he or she needs a complete assessment. Assessment is further separated into two phases: data collection and problem identification. As the nurse begins the task of gathering data, he or she may use three common techniques: interviews, observation, and physical examinations. The format for the collection of a nursing history varies among organizations. A usable nursing history should identify the patient's perception and expectations related to his or her illness, hospitalization, and care. Information should include demographic data, the patient's understanding of the illness, usual daily patterns, social and cultural history, ability to cope with problems, and ability to meet his or her own personal needs.

## Scope of assessment

Documented guidelines (policies and job descriptions, for instance) need to be in place to define the assessment activities that clinical disciplines within the hospital's settings perform. Standards are in place for the physicians and nurses specifically, but for other disciplines, the hospital must determine their expectations regarding patient assessment. In addition to a policy, an organization may have a multidisciplinary patient assessment admission form that is complete and concise in its documentation and allows caregivers from other disciplines to use the data collected from physicians and nurses upon admission.

## Assessment of patient's nursing care needs

In all settings that provide nursing care, an RN assesses the patient's nursing care needs and has a legal responsibility to analyze and evaluate the data collected for patients who receive nursing care. The RN must conclude whether additional assessment or intervention is necessary. Other qualified nursing staff members may perform data collection but not to the extent where the data are analyzed and a care plan is established.

Only an RN can analyze the assessment data and formulate a nursing diagnosis. To confirm data col-

 **Evidence-Based Falls Prevention, Second Edition**

lected by others and ensure that all necessary aspects of the patient's condition and needs have been assessed, the RN must directly observe the patient.

An organization's assessment policy should state that the RN is responsible for assessing the patient's need for nursing care on admission to any department in which nursing care is provided. The RN's job description will define the scope of assessment.

The surveyor will conduct a record review and may examine the organization's patient assessment policy. A surveyor may ask the following question during an interview with the staff: "What level of licensure does your organization require of the staff members who perform the initial patient assessment?"

# Clinical assessment review and insights to care of patients with specific needs

### Functional assessments

One healthcare objective is to improve or maintain the patient's functional abilities and overall quality of life. The functional assessment helps determine the patient's current level of functioning. Clinicians may then plan care to achieve improvement in the patient's functioning level. Functional assessments have resulted in extended life, less hospitalization, lowered medical costs, and improved functional status. A functional assessment measures the patient's ability to care for him or herself—to perform activities of daily living (ADLs). Patients should be recognized as at risk for falls when impairments in ADLs are identified. Determining the reason for the loss of function and when it occurred helps to identify the underlying cause and the potential for reversing the condition.

ADLs are divided into several levels. Basic activities of daily living involve performing personal care independently, such as feeding, being continent, transferring, toileting, dressing, and bathing. Instrumental activities of daily living are tasks necessary for independent functioning in the community, such as cooking, cleaning, doing laundry, shopping, using the telephone, taking medicines, and managing money.

During the initial assessment, screen the patient for risks to functional problems. Though all patients admitted to rehabilitation services should have received a functional assessment, many hospitals make the mistake of limiting the initial functional assessment to only these rehab patients.

Rather, the screen must be performed on all patients to determine who needs referral for rehabilitation services. Risk indicators identify patients who need further assessment by physical therapy (PT), occupational therapy (OT), or speech therapy (ST) disciplines, as applicable. Rehabilitation professionals identify these risk indicators. Physicians must write an order for any referrals for PT, OT, or ST. Therefore, consult a physician when a patient has a positive indicator during the functional screen that identifies the need for further assessment. The functional screen contains the following four elements:

- Risk indicators
- How many, or to what degree, indicators must be present
- Action taken when a risk is present
- Documentation of the action that occurred

The surveyor will conduct a medical record review to monitor that screening assessments are performed within 24 hours of admission. If a further assessment was indicated, the surveyor will check that the appropriate staff completed the rehabilitation assessment within the time frame specified in the organization's policy.

Include the functional assessment on the organization's multidisciplinary initial patient assessment form. A standardized flow sheet or checklist will ensure that the charting is complete. Figure 2.1 is one example of a functional assessment tool.

---

| **FIGURE 2.1** | **Functional assessment tool** |
|---|---|

**Physical therapy**

❐ PT consult needed

| | | |
|---|---|---|
| History of falls | ❐ Yes | ❐ No |
| Difficulty with mobility; unsteady gait, vertigo, dyspnea | ❐ Yes | ❐ No |
| Difficulty using assistive devices; assistive device used _____ | ❐ Yes | ❐ No |
| Loss of strength or paralysis | ❐ Yes | ❐ No |
| Acute muscle pain, cramps, or stiffness | ❐ Yes | ❐ No |

**Occupational therapy**

❐ OT consult needed

BADL able to perform:                                    IADL able to perform:

| | | | | | | |
|---|---|---|---|---|---|---|
| Bathing | ❐ Yes | ❐ No | Cooking | ❐ Yes | ❐ No |
| Feeding | ❐ Yes | ❐ No | Cleaning | ❐ Yes | ❐ No |
| Dressing | ❐ Yes | ❐ No | Laundry | ❐ Yes | ❐ No |
| Toileting | ❐ Yes | ❐ No | Shopping | ❐ Yes | ❐ No |
| Transferring | ❐ Yes | ❐ No | Driving | ❐ Yes | ❐ No |

**Speech therapy**

❐ ST consult needed

| | | |
|---|---|---|
| Difficulty with speech | ❐ Yes | ❐ No |
| Difficulty with swallowing | ❐ Yes | ❐ No |

❐ Fallprevention program initiated          ❐ Physician notified of functional screen results

Date: _____     RN signature _____

## Interdisciplinary patient care in action

### *Establishment of interdisciplinary plan of care*

As mentioned earlier, all patients must have an assessment completed by an RN within 24 hours of admission to determine their need for nursing care.

Screening assessments are also completed as part of this initial assessment process, and they determine the patient's need for in-depth assessments by nutrition, rehabilitation (PT/OT/speech-language pathology), and discharge planning staff. Patients are also screened for the possible presence of abuse or neglect, with referral to the appropriate discipline/agency for an in-depth assessment, if signs indicate such problems are present.

Hospitals expect their staff to develop a plan of care for patients to address any identified needs following this initial assessment and any subsequent reassessments. When only one discipline completes an assessment, it is solely this discipline that is involved in developing and implementing the patient plan of care.

Nursing will always perform an assessment for patients who are admitted, so the initial patient plan of care reflects problems identified by this discipline. At the time of admission, nursing is the only discipline, other than physicians, involved in the care of the patient. For some patients, this status continues throughout their entire stay. But for other patients, additional disciplines are asked to become involved in the care of the patient. This request is made by direct physician order, by medical staff–approved protocol, or as a result of the screening assessments completed by the RN at the time of nursing's initial assessment.

When nonnursing disciplines complete assessments, they often identify additional patient problems. It is expected that there will be a mechanism by which these additional disciplines' assessment and reassessment findings will be shared so that the list of patient problems reflects the results of assessments by all disciplines involved in the care of the patient.

It is important to remember that not all assessments lead to identification of patient problems. Some patients only require care that is of a routine nature. This care can be provided entirely through the use of protocols/standards of care or practice guidelines. These are established care or practice requirements. Even patients with identified individual problems frequently have a part of their care provided through the use of protocols.

Think of these protocols as the operating system in your computer. You don't see it, but it's always at work. These protocols are called the "routine care"—getting an IV, needing help with personal hygiene, or using a vent—which any patient can expect to receive. The bottom portion of Figure 2.2 is an example of a tool that can be used to document the care provided through protocols.

 **Evidence-Based Falls Prevention, Second Edition**

**FIGURE 2.2** — **Problem list**

| Problems | Initial Priority | | Revised Priority | | Revised Priority | | Revised Priority | |
|---|---|---|---|---|---|---|---|---|
| | Discipline | # | Discipline | # | Discipline | # | Discipline | # |
| | | | | | | | | |
| | | | | | | | | |
| | | | | | | | | |
| | | | | | | | | |
| | | | | | | | | |
| | | | | | | | | |
| | | | | | | | | |

No priority issues identified. Care planned through use of protocols/standards only ☐

| Protocol/Standard | 7-3 | 3-11 | 11-7 | 7-3 | 3-11 | 11-7 | 7-3 | 3-11 | 11-7 | 7-3 | 3-11 | 11-7 |
|---|---|---|---|---|---|---|---|---|---|---|---|---|
| Date | | | | | | | | | | | | |
| Physiological Monitoring | | | | | | | | | | | | |
| Elimination | | | | | | | | | | | | |
| Peripheral I.V. Therapy | | | | | | | | | | | | |
| Fall Injury Prevention | | | | | | | | | | | | |
| Alteration in Skin/Tissue Integrity | | | | | | | | | | | | |
| Oxygen management | | | | | | | | | | | | |
| Foley Management | | | | | | | | | | | | |
| Alteration in Nutrition | | | | | | | | | | | | |
| Remote Telemetry Monitoring | | | | | | | | | | | | |
| Post Operative Management | | | | | | | | | | | | |
| Hypo/Hyperthermia Management | | | | | | | | | | | | |
| Anticoagulant Therapy Management | | | | | | | | | | | | |
| Central line Management | | | | | | | | | | | | |
| Hygiene | | | | | | | | | | | | |
| PCA | | | | | | | | | | | | |
| Mechanical Ventilation | | | | | | | | | | | | |

| Initial | First, Last Name and Title | Initial | First, Last Name and Title | Initial | First, Last Name & Title |
|---|---|---|---|---|---|

Of course, an existing protocol/standard/guideline must already be present for this to apply.

In keeping with the computer analogy, the individualized plan of care is similar to when a warning box pops up on your computer screen. That warning box appears on your screen because something in your operating system has said, "Here is something to which you need to pay attention." Whatever prompts the warning must be added to the patient's individualized plan of care.

Some assessments, most often those related to "false positive" screening assessments, indicate no problem at all. Other assessments may indicate the presence of a problem that is inappropriate to begin addressing at the time it is identified. Yet other assessments reveal problems that the patient is uninterested in pursuing, such as weight loss to counter obesity.

The analogy for these situations is one with which many of you are already familiar. It is where one physician asks another physician to see the patient and offer additions to the medical plan of care, if needed. In some cases, the consulting physician completes the assessment of the patient and identifies no other problems or has no additional thoughts on patient management. The consult note usually ends with a statement such as "Thank you for this interesting consult. I have nothing to add to the patient's plan of care at this time. Call me if anything changes, and I will be glad to see the patient again."

The same possibility exists following an assessment by a nonnursing discipline. Assessment findings may be documented, but no problem may be identified. Or a problem could be identified, but there is no interest from the patient in addressing it, so the patient plan is not affected unless something changes (e.g., another assessment is requested and indicates a problem, or the patient changes his or her mind about addressing a problem).

## Documentation

Although nursing is only one segment of the healthcare team working with patients at risk of falling, nurses should maintain responsibility and accountability for coordinating and integrating the interdisciplinary plan of care.

The interdisciplinary plan of care should be maintained in a place mutually agreed upon by the clinical team so that all disciplines can document their evaluations of the patient's progress toward achieving his or her goals. If computerized documentation is utilized, all disciplines need access to each other's documentation at all times. Findings available to only one discipline, and plans maintained by disciplines in isolation of each other, defeat the intent of an interdisciplinary process of care delivery.

The interdisciplinary plan of care should be a working document used by all members of the clinical team to record identification and resolution of patient problems (see Figure 2.3). It should accompany the patient throughout hospitalization.

Members of the team may change as the patient progresses through the continuum of care, but the interdisciplinary plan of care should accompany the patient throughout the continuum and be used by all disciplines to guide the delivery of appropriate care to the patient, exchange information, hand off care, and document progress toward goal attainment.

| FIGURE 2.3 | | Interdisciplinary plan of care tool sample | | | | |
|---|---|---|---|---|---|---|

| Date | Init. | Patient Care Problem | Goal(s) or Outcome(s) | Date to be met | Interventions | Discipline(s) Responsible |
|---|---|---|---|---|---|---|
|  |  |  |  |  |  |  |

Discipline Responsible Key

| | | | | | |
|---|---|---|---|---|---|
| **CM** | Case Management | **P** | Pharmacy | **SLP** | Speech Language Pathology |
| **D** | Dietician | **PC** | Pastoral care | **SW** | Social Work |
| **N** | Nursing | **PT** | Physical Therapy | **O** | Other (Specify) |
| **OT** | Occupational Therapy | **RT** | Respiratory Therapy | | |

**Goal Evaluation**

Date _____     Goal # _____

☐ Goal Met
☐ Goal not met + Progress
　　☐ Continue, no change
　　☐ Goal Revised
　　☐ Interventions revised
☐ Goal not met – Progress
　　☐ Goal Revised
　　☐ Interventions revised

Date _____     Goal # _____

☐ Goal Met
☐ Goal not met + Progress
　　☐ Continue, no change
　　☐ Goal Revised
　　☐ Interventions revised
☐ Goal not met – Progress
　　☐ Goal Revised
　　☐ Interventions revised

　　　　© 2007 HCPro, Inc.　　　**Evidence-Based Falls Prevention, Second Edition**

# Problem identification

Assessments are completed in order to determine whether patient problems exist. When only the nursing staff has completed assessments and identified patient problems, the assessment will reflect problems identified by only this discipline. In this case, nursing alone will prioritize the identified problems and develop a plan of care to address those patients needing immediate attention.

But many patients have assessments completed by more than one discipline. As a result, problems may be identified in addition to those identified by nursing. Because of this, there must be a way to share assessment findings from the various disciplines that completed assessments so that the complete list of patient problems can be developed.

Only then can decisions be made as to which problems have the highest priority. What had been the most pressing problems may be less critical as additional problems are identified and the list expands. This list will usually change over the course of a patient's hospital stay, as new problems are identified and others are resolved or controlled. The problem list may be an actual recorded list or just a concept that is reflected in the plan of care at any point in time.

Figure 2.4 is a tool developed by a 250-bed community hospital for members of the clinical team to use to identify and communicate problems to other members of the team who are unable to meet face to face.

The clinical team needs to make the following decisions regarding how identified problems are assigned a priority status:

- Will prioritization be done by the RN alone, or will all those disciplines that identified problems have a voice?

- Will the team identifying problems actually vote on this prioritization and assign a priority number to the problems, or will this be done in concept only?

- Will prioritization occur each time the problem list is reviewed/revised?

| FIGURE 2.4 | Interdisciplinary team conference assessment |
|---|---|

Age/Diagnosis _____ Date: _____

**Case Management/Discharge Planning:** ☐ **No needs identified at this time**
☐ Assess Needs ☐ Home Health ☐ Rehabilitation ☐ SNF ☐ Rest Home ☐ DME ☐ Financial Assistance
Pre-Adm. DME/Services _____ ☐ Other Community Resource: _____
Signature: _____

**Nutrition:** ☐ To Evaluate ☐ Diet Assessment ☐ Snacks ☐ Calorie Count ☐ TPN/TF ☐ Education ☐ Evaluation completed
☐ Bottlefeeding ☐ Breastfeeding ☐ Other _____ Signature: _____

**Rehabilitation:**
Physical Therapy ☐ To Evaluate ☐ ROM ☐ Transfers ☐ Gait ☐ Exercise ☐ Balance/coordination ☐ Pt./Family education
☐ Other: _____
☐ WBAT ☐ PWB ☐ TDWB ☐ NWB
Asst. Device: _____ CPM _____
☐ No progress ☐ Slow progress ☐ Steady progress
Signature: _____

Speech Therapy ☐ To Evaluate ☐ Speech Therapy ☐ Speech/Lang. Tx. ☐ Dysphagia Tx. ☐ Pt./Family Education
☐ Cognitive Lang Tx. ☐ Home program instruction ☐ Diet consistency: _____
☐ Other: _____
☐ No progress ☐ Slow progress ☐ Steady progress
Signature: _____

Occupational Therapy ☐ To Evaluate ☐ ADL's ☐ Therapeutic Exercise ☐ Coordination ☐ Cognitive retaining ☐ Pt/Family ed.
☐ Visual-perceptual skills ☐ Sensory re-education ☐ Stress management ☐ Energy conservation
☐ Adaptive Equipment ☐ Other _____
☐ No progress ☐ Slow progress ☐ Steady progress
Signature: _____

**Pharmacy:** PO Meds: ☐ Yes ☐ No ☐ Afebrile
IV Meds/Antibiotics Appropriate: ☐ Yes ☐ No ☐ Routine Meds
Dose Appropriate: ☐ Yes ☐ No Other: _____
Medication Duplications: ☐ Yes ☐ No _____
Signature: _____

**Pastoral Care/Patient Representative Counseling:**
☐ Grief/Death ☐ Religious ☐ Pt/Family Complaint ☐ Pt/Family Advocacy ☐ Living Will/Healthcare POA
☐ Psychological ☐ Pre and Post Opt. needs ☐ Terminal Illness ☐ Personal Concerns
☐ Educational Needs Assessment ☐ Other _____
Signature: _____

**Nursing Interventions:**
☐ High Risk for Falls ☐ High Risk for Skin Break Down ☐ Wound Care ☐ Special Bed ☐ Restraints
☐ Alternatives to restraints _____ ☐ Pt/Family Education ☐ High Risk for Aspiration
☐ Other _____
Signature: _____

**Other:** ☐ First Step ☐ Diabetic Teaching ☐ Lactation Consultant ☐ Mental Health ☐ Ostomy Teaching
☐ Health Dept. F/U ☐ Interpreter Services ☐ Postnatal Ed. ☐ DSS F/U
Recorder: _____

**ADDRESSOGRAPH**

Union Regional Medical Center
P.O. Box 5003
Monroe, North Carolina 28111

URMC-0368 (10/98)

**Evidence-Based Falls Prevention, Second Edition**

## *Resolved problems*

Problems should be eliminated from the plan of care as they are resolved (i.e., when the patient meets his or her goals) or when it is clear that the problems cannot be resolved during admission, in which case a plan is created to hand off the problem to another caregiver in the continuum of care (assuming continuation is needed). For example, a resolved problem might be the attainment of the patient's goal to stand from a seated position, walk eight feet, and return to a seated position in the same chair within 20 seconds (the "Eight-Foot Get Up and Go" test, as mentioned in Chapter 5).

Also consider that there might be situations in which the definitive goal is not met, but progress has been made and the team (or nursing, if it is the only discipline involved in the care of the patient) determines the problem to be controlled (i.e., the goal has been met as well as it can be).

In the preceding scenario, for example, suppose the patient performed the "Eight-Foot Get Up and Go" test in 30 seconds instead of the goal of 20 seconds due to persistent body sway and muscle weakness. The goal was not attained, but the patient improved from the first tested time of 40 seconds. The goal of 20 seconds might be unrealistic for this patient. So, even though the underlying problem was not resolved and the goal was not met, the team could determine that a time of 30 seconds is as much progress as the patient can make. This would eliminate the problem from the plan.

# CHAPTER 3:

## Risk factors for falls

# Risk factors for falls

## Learning objectives

After reading this chapter, the participant should be able to:

- Define a fall
- Identify several nonmodifiable intrinsic fall risk factors
- List examples of modifiable risk factors

## Introduction

A fall can be defined as any sudden, unintentional change in position that causes an individual to land at a lower level, on an object, on the floor, or on the ground. If you find a patient on the floor, therefore, you may assume that a fall has occurred. If a patient loses his or her balance and someone lowers him or her to the floor, a fall has occurred. Falls can be witnessed or not witnessed, and fallers may or may not be able to explain what caused a fall. However, The Joint Commission stated in 2006 that each organization needs to define what it considers to be a patient/resident fall[1].

People fall for many different reasons, and most falls have more than one cause. Patients usually fall during routine activities, such as walking, standing, or changing position. Approximately 50% of falls result primarily from extrinsic factors in the environment. Other falls result mostly from factors intrinsic to the patient, such as physical conditions or medication use. Although one of these two factors may be the primary cause of the fall, most often the fall is the result of complex interactions of several factors, both intrinsic and extrinsic. The rate of falls increases proportionately with the number of cognitive and functional impairments and risk factors present in an individual or population.

The first step to reducing falls is identifying the factors that put patients at risk. When we recognize those things that increase a person's likelihood of falling, we can calculate each individual's fall risk and plan appropriate interventions. As you review these risk factors, keep in mind that the more risk factors a person has, the higher the likelihood that a fall will occur.

## Nonmodifiable intrinsic risk factors

Several nonmodifiable intrinsic traits are potential risk factors for falls. Statistically, factors such as age, gender, race, and past history of falling increase the likelihood that a patient will fall. Although we cannot change these characteristics, we can recognize the danger for patients who possess these traits and plan their care accordingly. Figure 3.1 examines some of these traits.

| FIGURE 3.1 | Nonmodifiable intrinsic fall risk factors |
| --- | --- |

**Gender**
- Women fall more often and are almost three times more likely than men to require hospitalization for a fall-related injury

**Race**
- White people have the highest risk of falling
- White men have the highest rate of fall-related deaths, followed by white women

**Age**
- Falls are the most common cause of injuries and hospital admissions due to trauma for people aged 65 and older
- More than 60% of people who die from falls are aged 75 and older
- The risk of falling increases exponentially with age, and the chance that a fall will cause a severe injury that requires hospitalization increases significantly with age
- Fifty percent to 75% of the residents in long-term care facilities fall each year

**History of falls**
- A previous fall doubles or triples the likelihood of an older adult falling again
- A family history of falls increases an older adult's chance of falling

Although these intrinsic risk factors are not modifiable, they can help us recognize which patients are at high risk for falling. For instance, a 76-year-old white female who has fallen before is in a very high-risk fall category and requires aggressive interventions.

### *Other physical risk factors*

Two of the most frequently documented risk factors for falls are mobility problems and poor health status. Often these two factors coexist, with poor health causing mobility problems and vice versa. Figure 3.2 lists medical conditions that research has shown to increase fall risk.

| FIGURE 3.2 | Medical conditions that increase fall risk |
|---|---|

- Having more than one chronic disease of any kind
- Vascular disorders, such as:
  - History of stroke
  - Hypertension
  - Hypotension, orthostatic hypotension, and postprandial hypotension
  - Neurocardiovascular instability (cardioinhibitory carotid sinus hypersensitivity or carotid sinus syndrome)
  - Cardiovascular disorders
- Neuromuscular disorders, such as:
  - Parkinson's disease
  - Multiple sclerosis
  - Others, such as Huntington's chorea
- Musculoskeletal disorders, such as:
  - Arthritis
  - Hip fractures
  - Osteoporosis
  - Amputation
  - Foot disorders and deformities
- Neurological disorders, such as:
  - Seizure disorder
  - Peripheral neuropathies
  - Dementia
- Sensory loss, such as:
  - Poor visual acuity
  - Diminished visual contrast sensitivity
  - Flattened visual depth perception
  - Slow visual reflexes (visual reflexes help control posture and balance)
  - Diminished hearing, which affects balance
- Lung diseases such as chronic obstructive pulmonary disease (COPD) that cause poor oxygenation of cells
- Bowel or urinary urgency or incontinence, which can cause a person to move too quickly

Mobility problems may exist regardless of whether medical disorders are present. Some of these difficulties may be due to a modifiable characteristic, while others may exist because of an illness or disability. They include:

- Gait abnormalities.

- Poor balance.

- Postural instability or impairment of gait and balance. Patients with combined gait and balance difficulties are three times more likely to fall than those with normal gait and balance.

- Lower-body weakness, particularly leg weakness. Some studies indicate a five-fold increased risk of falling for individuals with weak legs. Researchers have documented severely weak ankles in the elderly with a history of falling.

- General weakness.

- Inadequate overall muscle strength, particularly trunk-muscle weakness. The trunk muscles maintain balance.

- Joint and muscle stiffness and reduction in range of motion. There is some evidence that older adults with a history of falling may have a smaller range of motion in comparison to those who don't have a history. Reduced range of motion could interfere with movement control and balance.

## Modifiable risk factors

### Lifestyle risk factors

Modifiable physical risk factors include those related to a patient's lifestyle choices. Although we can reduce the potential for falling and for fall-related injuries by changing these lifestyle characteristics, patients need support and encouragement to help them change lifelong, ingrained habits. Lifestyle risk factors include the following:

- Inadequate nutrition, which increases the risk of falling and also the chance of serious injury from falls
    - Inadequate calcium and vitamin D intake leads to low bone mass
    - Inadequate protein and calorie intake leads to low muscle mass and weakness

- Excessive alcohol intake, whether acute or chronic, which contributes to a variety of short- and long-term problems with balance, nutrition, weakness, and movement control

- Inactivity, which causes deterioration in muscle strength, bone mass, and joint flexibility

- Loss of strength and flexibility which leads to loss of confidence and fear of falling

- Lower bone mass which makes injury more likely when a fall occurs

- Smoking, which leads to poor cellular oxygenation and low bone mass

## Medication

A major modifiable risk factor is the medications patients take. Patients who take more than four medications are statistically more likely to fall than those who take fewer drugs. Up to 42% of people aged 70 and older take four or more medications. As the total number of drugs taken increases, so does the risk of falling. Polypharmacy also increases the risk of harmful drug interactions and decreases compliance with appropriate medications, providing an even greater reason for prescribing as few drugs as medically possible.

People who take psychotropic medications, including sedatives, antidepressants, neurologic/antieplipetics, and other drugs that act on the central nervous system also have a high risk of falling. Sedatives slow reaction times and reduce awareness of the environment, both of which can increase a patient's risk of falling.

Many central nervous system–active drugs can cause hypotension in susceptible people, which can lead to lightheadedness and unsteadiness. Neuroleptic drugs can cause hypotension as well as visual blurring and drug-induced Parkinson's disease. Benzodiazepines such as Valium cause sedation and impair postural stability.

In addition to too many medications and the wrong kinds of medications, excessive dosages are a risk factor for falls. Since drug elimination is slower in the elderly, doses that are too high or medications that are taken for an unnecessarily long period of time often contribute to falls. People on benzodiazepines who fell, for example, were found to have higher serum concentrations of the drug than those who took the medication but did not fall.[2] Some researchers believe that medications are responsible for as many as 20% of all falls.

## Depression medications

Depressive symptoms can include impaired motor coordination and response time, which increase the risk of falls. Depression also increases the risk for osteoporosis, possibly because of changes in adrenal function. Despite the many negative consequences of depression, including falls, it is frequently misdiagnosed or inappropriately treated.

Many people are treated for depression with tricyclic antidepressants (TCAs) or selective serotonin reuptake inhibitors (SSRIs). Treatment for depression is problematic where falls are concerned, because the medications commonly prescribed for depressive symptoms are psychotropic drugs, which are major risk factors for falling in the elderly. A number of studies of the elderly have found a significant increase in the risk of falls or fractures with the use of either type of antidepressant.[3] Additionally, the side effects of certain psychotropic medications may increase the risk of falls to any patient population.

When prescribing antidepressants, physicians should start medications at a low dose and increase them slowly. It is important to review concomitant medications and assess the potential for drug interactions. All other risk factors for falls should be modified where possible when antidepressant use is necessary to keep fall risk to a minimum in spite of the medications.

The Beers' criteria is a list of medications that seniors should not take because of potentially serious harmful effects.[4] In a review of more than 8,100 outpatient visits made by seniors to doctors' offices and hospitals over a five-year period, 7.8% included an elderly person receiving one or more prescriptions from the list of Beers' criteria medications to avoid.

Elderly women over age 65 were twice as likely to receive an inappropriate prescription as elderly men. The risk of getting an unsafe medication was higher for patients who took several medications compared to those who took fewer medications.[5] Many of the medications on the Beers' criteria are unsafe for the elderly at least in part because of sedative/anticholinergic properties that put the

**Evidence-Based Falls Prevention, Second Edition**

patient at risk for falling. The key here is to administer a complete review of medications that a patient is on—medication reconciliation in relationship to fall risk is important.

## Psychological and cognitive risk factors

Patients' behavior and habits may put them at risk for falls, including:

- A strong desire for independence, making patients reluctant to ask for assistance or use assistive devices
- Unwillingness to comply with instructions or a regimen
- Fear of falling or loss of confidence in physical abilities

### *Dementia*

People with dementia present a particular problem where falls are concerned. People with cognitive impairment are more likely to wander, become agitated, and have perceptual difficulties. Perception of dimensionality and place in space (proprioception) also may be impaired. Individuals in middle and late stages of degenerative dementias have lost the ability to perceive in three dimensions.

Those with dementia are three times more likely to sustain a fracture from a fall, and the majority of fractures occur in the neck of the femur. Nursing home residents with dementia who sustain a hip fracture have a 50% higher mortality rate at one year than those without dementia. Dementia sufferers who fall are five times more likely to be institutionalized than dementia sufferers who do not fall.

There are some risk factors that are specific to patients with cognitive impairment, as well as risk factors shared with other older adults that have greater significance for these patients. While dementia can occur in younger people, the incidence increases with age. In the United States, 1.2 million people suffer from severe depression, and 2.5 million battle a moderate form of the disease. Of those sufferers, 0.5% are between the ages of 60 and 64, and 3.2% are between the ages of 80 and 90.[6] Risk factors specific to older people with dementia include:

- Wandering

- Agitation

- Perceptual difficulties, such as:
    - Lack of visuospatial awareness
    - Flattened visual field

- Lack of fear or caution/poor judgment

- Balance impairments, such as:
    - Increased double support time (the time during which both feet are in contact with the ground) while walking, which indicates greater instability.
    - Increased sway path. A larger sway path (postural sway measures give information relative to postural steadiness; a larger sway magnitude is related to greater postural unsteadiness) indicates more swaying when walking, producing greater postural unsteadiness.
    - Increased unsteadiness.
    - Impaired one/two leg balance, eyes open/closed.

- Gait impairments, such as:
    - Slower walking speed
    - Reduced step frequency
    - Shorter step length
    - Increased postural flexion

Risk factors shared with people without dementia that have particular relevance for those with dementia include:

- Postural instability (gait and balance impairment)
- Medication, especially psychotropics
- Neurocardiovascular instability, especially orthostatic hypotension (higher prevalence in people with dementia)
- Environmental fall hazards
- Visual impairment

There is some evidence that people with vascular dementia are at greater risk for falls than those with Alzheimer's disease. Those with vascular dementia have more marked gait abnormalities, significantly slower velocity, and shorter step length than those with Alzheimer's.

Most falls in patients with dementia have multiple causes. One study identified a median of four risk factors for falls in each older subject with cognitive impairment.[7] The most common of these were:

- Postural instability; gait and balance impairment
- Environmental hazards
- Medication
- Neurocardiovascular instability, particularly orthostatic hypotension

## *Fear of falling*

A condition variously described as "space phobia," "post-fall syndrome," or "fear of falling" has been documented in 21%–61% of elderly people.[8] Among those who have actually fallen, the prevalence is 32%–83%.[9] Fear of falling leads to reduced independence and self-imposed restrictions. Among older adults who report this fear, up to 70% admit that they avoid activities because of it. Activity restriction can lead to muscle atrophy, porous bones, and poor balance, which is, in itself, a risk factor for falls.[10] Activity restriction can produce social isolation, which contributes to depression, another fall risk factor.[11]

Several studies have connected fear of falling with depression and anxiety. Depression and anxiety scores were the major predictors of chronic dizziness in a study of older people, and the dizziness was significantly correlated with fear of falling. Another study discovered that those with post-fall syndrome were more likely to score above 11 on the Geriatric Depression Scale, which is the cutoff point to indicate mild or more severe depression.

Individuals with some of the following factors have a greater fear of falling:

- Older age
- Female
- Experience of previous falls
- Falls requiring medical attention
- Falls resulting in fracture
- Falls that occur in circumstances other than a slip or trip
- Delay getting up after a fall
- Decreased mobility
- Poor performance on tests of balance
- Chronic dizziness

- Higher levels of pain
- Living alone or having few social contacts
- Poor life satisfaction
- Frailty and the need for assistance
- Use of an assistive ambulatory device
- Poor vision
- Poor health
- Restriction in activities of daily living

## *Balance and inner ear problems*

A major reason for falls is poor balance. The complicated human balance system is impacted by vision, the inner ear, and the central nervous system. Our inner ears sense when we are in motion and give the central nervous system information it needs to adjust posture and exert muscular control to keep us upright. The inner ear perceives gravity as well as motion, helping to make the necessary accommodations to gravitational forces.[12]

Any disorder of the inner ear can impair balance, including infections and earwax buildup. Earwax buildup is fairly common, causing symptoms in as many as 12.5% of the population by some reports.[13] Circumstances that increase the likelihood of earwax accumulation include a narrow, hairy inner ear canal; use of a hearing aid; being elderly; or having chronic inflammation of the external canal.

A sedentary lifestyle causes another inner ear problem. As we move around, we keep the fluid in the inner ear active and viable. Those who don't move around much lose this benefit. The fluid in the inner ear is a crucial part of our balance system, so those with inadequate inner ear fluid may have impaired balance.

## *Cardiovascular risk factors*

Cardiovascular risk factors may account for as many as 77% of unexplained or recurrent falls and falls occurring with an unexplained loss of consciousness. If a patient falls without attempting to stop the fall or self-rescue, consider a cardiovascular cause. Fallers with an intrinsic cardiac cause have a higher rate of mortality than those with other causes.

According to several studies, up to one in three older people who experience an unexplained fall may have carotid sinus syndrome, also called cardioinhibitory carotid sinus hypersensitivity, which is treatable with a pacemaker. Some researchers propose that proper treatment could prevent up to 70% of falls and state that carotid sinus hypersensitivity should be considered in all patients who experience nonaccidental falls.[14] Carotid sinus syndrome causes amnesia, so the patient will not remember blacking out prior to falling. If a patient cannot tell you why he or she fell, a cardiac or syncopal episode is likely. Figure 3.3 lists other cardiovascular risk factors for falls.

## FIGURE 3.3 · Cardiovascular causes of falls

- Vasovagal syncope

- Situational syncopes (caused by coughing, sneezing, micturition, defecation, gastrointestinal stimulation, Valsalva, deglutition, diving reflex)

- Cardiac abnormalities, such as:
  - Supraventricular arrhythmias
  - Ventricular arrhythmias
  - Structural abnormalities, for example:
    - Valvular stenosis
    - Myocardial infarction
    - Aortic dissection
    - Tamponade
    - Cardiomyopathy

- Pulmonary embolism

- Cerebral syncope

- Transient ischemic attacks

- Migraine

- Subclavian steal syndrome

# Extrinsic risk factors

Environmental hazards are a major cause of falls, including:

- **Furniture arrangement**, as arrangements can sometimes block pathways. This can be a problem in any care environment.

- **Floors** that are too slick and changes in flooring types or levels from one room to another have all been responsible for falls, as well as wrinkled, torn, or uneven flooring of any kind. Scattered rugs without secure anchoring may slip and cause someone to trip.

- **Lighting** that is too low is a risk factor for falls, as is lighting that is too bright, creates glare, or distorts the way objects look (as can happen with colored lights).

- **Trailing cords or hoses** from electrical devices, vacuum cleaners, or floor washers cause falls.

- **Temperature** affects fall risk in two ways. People with orthostatic hypotension should avoid hot environments, as the heat can result in vasodilation. For example, people with multiple sclerosis often find that heat exacerbates their illness. On the other hand, cold weather can make stiff joints even more inflexible. A moderate indoor temperature is best to prevent the effect of temperature extremes on either end of the spectrum.

- **New, unfamiliar surroundings** cause falls. For example, research shows that the incidence of falls is highest in the first week a person moves to a new environment.[15]

- **Clothing that is too long** is often responsible for falls. Skirts and pants that touch the floor are fall hazards.

- **Footwear** is a major risk factor for falls. Thick, rubbery soles catch easily on carpet and cause tripping. Socks without treads can easily cause a fall on a slick floor.

     **Evidence-Based Falls Prevention, Second Edition**

# References

1. The Joint Commission. *www.jointcommission.org/NR/rdonlyres/D4844675-25D7-4B5B-A47D-C549D939F9E5/0/07_NPSG_FAQs_9.pdf*. Visited on 8/14/07.

2. Ryynanen, O.P., Kivela, S.L., Honkanen, R, Laippala, P., and Saano, V. (1993). "Medications and chronic diseases as risk factors for falling injuries in the elderly." *The Scandinavian Journal of Social Medicine 1993;21:264–271.*

3. Liu, B. (2003). "Relationship between antidepressants and the risk of falls." *Geriatrics & Aging July/August 2003 6:(7):45–47.*

4. Beers, M.H. (1997). "Explicit criteria for determining potentially inappropriate medication use by the elderly." *Archives of Internal Medicine 157:1531–1536.*

5. Goulding M. R. (2004). "Inappropriate medication prescribing for elderly ambulatory care patients." *Archives of Internal Medicine 164:(3):305–312.*

6. Knight, A. L. "Dementia." Griffith's 5-Minute Clinical Consult: A Reference for Clinicians. *www.5mcc.com/Assets/SUMMARY/TP0250.html.*

7. (2003). "Multifactorial intervention after a fall in older people with cognitive impairment and dementia presenting to the accident and emergency department: Randomised controlled trial." *British Medical Journal;* 326:73–75.

8. (2003). Gagnon, and Flint, A. J. (2003). "Fear of falling in the elderly." *Geriatrics & Aging;* (6):7:15–17.

9. Vellas, B.J., Wayne, S.J., Romero, L.J., et al. (1997). "Fear of falling and restriction of mobility in elderly fallers." *Age and Aging;* 26:189–93.

10. Maki, B.E., Holliday, P.J., and Topper AK. (1991). "Fear of falling and postural performance in the elderly." *Journal of Gerontol;* 46:M123–131.

11. Howland, J., Peterson E.W., Levin, W.C., et al. (1993). "Fear of falling among the community-dwelling elderly." *Journal of Aging and Health*; 5:229–243.

12. "Cleaning earwax: Why you shouldn't play it by ear." Urkin, J., Gazala, E., and Bar-David, Y. Contemporary Pediatrics Archive February 2004. *www.modernmedicine.com/modernmedicine/article/articledetail.jsp?id=108008*

13. (1990). Sharp, J.F., Wilson, J.A., Ross, L., et al. (1990). "Ear wax removal: A survey of current practice." *British Medical Journal*; 301:1251.

14. Kenny, R. A. M., Richardson, D. A., Steen, N., Bexton, R. S., Shaw, F. E., and Bond J. "Carotid sinus syndrome: A modifiable risk factor for nonaccidental falls in older adults" (SAFE PACE). *International Journal of the American College of Cardiology*, 38:(5):1491–1496.

15. Klein, K. and Ritzel, D. O. "Falls pose a serious threat to the elderly." *www.nsc.org/issues/ifalls/falthreat.htm*. NSC Issue—Falls in the Home.

**Evidence-Based Falls Prevention, Second Edition**

# CHAPTER 4:

# Modifications based on risk factor identification: Preventing falls

# 4

# Modifications based on risk factor identification: Preventing falls

## Learning objectives

After reading this chapter, the participant should be able to:

- List functional risk factor modifications
- Describe recommendations for preventing falls in the cognitively impaired
- List specific medical conditions responsible for falls that are often overlooked

## Introduction

With the national focus on fall prevention, it is important to concentrate on the full patient population. Proactive assessment of all patients will likely assist in decreasing the incidence of increased lengths of stay, rehabilitation as a result of falls, and increased costs associated with falls. An examination of the many risk factors for falls makes it clear why fall rates are so high. Every patient potentially can be at risk to fall during a hospitalization. After the initial assessment, the next step is to determine what kinds of interventions and modifications can lessen the impact of these risk factors.

Nothing can be done to change nonmodifiable risk factors such as age, gender, race, and history. However, chronic diseases can be managed to reduce those side effects that make patients more prone to falling, and environments can be monitored and modified to remove environmental hazards.

# Functional risk factor modifications

### Nutrition

Nutrition has a significant impact on the general health and well-being of patients. Older people have a greater need for nutrient-dense foods, since they often consume fewer calories than do younger adults. The food they eat must be full of beneficial elements besides calories, particularly calcium, vitamin D, and vitamin C for bone mass and protein for muscle strength.

### Calcium and vitamin D intake

Researchers have found a positive correlation between vitamin D and calcium and musculoskeletal function in several studies. There was a decrease in body sway in ambulatory elderly women following two months of treatment with 800 IU of vitamin D a day and 1,200 mg of calcium a day and a reduction in falls within one year. A study of institutionalized elderly women revealed a 49% reduction in fall risk within 12 weeks of vitamin D and calcium supplementation in the same doses. These effects can be explained in part by the biological action of vitamin D on muscle tissue. Muscle weakness is a risk factor for structural joint damage, which in turn leads to disorders like osteoarthritis, a risk factor for falls.[1]

Vitamin D and calcium supplementation are successful not only in reducing falls but also in lowering fracture risk. The Nurses' Health Study in the United States found that women who consumed at least 500 IU of vitamin D per day had a 37% lower risk of hip fracture. Researchers attribute these effects to the benefit of both vitamin D and calcium on bone mineral density.[2]

### Alcohol

People at risk for falling should generally avoid alcohol. Alcohol consumption can result in vasodilation, a factor in orthostatic hypotension (OH), as well as dizziness, unsteady gait, impaired vision, impaired judgment, and sedation. In addition, alcohol often potentiates or otherwise interacts with the effects of medication in unpredictable ways.

### Orthostatic hypotension

Food intake can have a significant impact on people with OH. These individuals should have a liberal salt intake unless there are clinical contraindications, and they should drink plenty of fluids. Meals can cause postprandial OH, which is a decrease in systolic blood pressure of 20 mmHg or more within two hours after a meal. This type of hypotension is distinct from OH but may occur in conjunction with it. The exact mechanism is not known. If an individual shows clinical signs of

 **Evidence-Based Falls Prevention, Second Edition**

postprandial OH, smaller and more frequent meals are advised, with the biggest meal consumed in the evening. Caffeine has vasopressor effects and can help limit OH. Individuals who suffer from frequent OH should drink two cups of coffee with breakfast and lunch.

## Smoking

Smoking is an extremely difficult habit to break and often requires a doctor's assistance and medications to treat symptoms of nicotine withdrawal. Help and encourage any patient who is willing to make the effort to stop smoking. For those who are not, we must recognize that their habit has put them in a high-risk category for falls.

## Exercise

Exercise is a major topic in fall-prevention research. Exercise, even brisk walking, actually increases the risk of falls and injuries. A fear of falling will impact exercise, and loss of muscle tone and strength will impact person's ability to react to a fall. A number of studies on untargeted group exercises have failed to demonstrate a reduction in falls. However, exercise has many benefits such as improving balance control, confidence, and bone mass. Researchers believe the issue is not exercise itself, but finding the type of exercise programs most likely to provide the greatest benefits.

On the whole, there is sufficient evidence that exercise reduces the risk of falling when included as part of a multifactorial intervention program. Exercises that develop postural balance control are the most successful, although strength and flexibility development provide adjunct benefits that may reduce injuries. Figure 4.1 examines a number of exercise studies and their resultant effects on participants' fall rates. Because inpatient stays are generally brief, an exercise program is unrealistic. However, physical therapy and occupational therapy on a routine basis during an inpatient stay can assist patients at risk and help them develop, maintain, or improve their postural balance control.

The ability to maintain balance is critical to avoiding falls. Balance is dependent on a highly sophisticated neural system that integrates information about the body's orientation and motion from a variety of sensory sources. This information then directs the motor responses that keep the body upright. Continuous balance control is required for all actions, and if there is an unexpected challenge caused by a trip, the body must rapidly compensate with appropriate movements. With age, the decline in sensory function and musculoskeletal condition make this delicate balancing act more difficult. Although exercise may not be able to correct sensory deficits, it may improve the ability of the system to process and respond to sensory input.

| FIGURE 4.1 | Effective exercise programs tested in randomized controlled trials | | |
| --- | --- | --- | --- |

| Article, sample | Exercise intervention | Evidence of effectiveness |
| --- | --- | --- |
| Buchner et al.[3]<br>68–85 y/o with mild deficits in strength and balance | • Group sessions supervised for one hour, three days/week for 24–26 weeks, then self-supervised<br>• Strength training for upper and lower body using weight machines<br>• Endurance training using stationary bicycles, 30–35 min/session | • Exercises for strength, endurance, and strength plus endurance vs. no active intervention reduced time to first fall<br>• Falls monitored for up to 25 months |
| Campbell et al.[4]<br>Women 80 years and older<br>Robertson et al.[5]<br>Men and women 75 years and older | • Program individually prescribed by physiotherapist or nurse trained and supervised by physio-therapist. Strength and balance training.<br>• Set of progressive, moderate intensity leg muscle strengthening and balance retraining exercises. Ankle cuff weights used for resistance.<br>• Exercises took 30 minutes, three times weekly; walking plan, 30 minutes at least twice a week. | • Exercise vs. social visits reduced falls by 32% at one year in research setting, and by 31% over two years<br>• Exercise vs. usual care reduced falls by 46% at one year in home health service setting<br>• Further evidence from a controlled trial in multiple centers in general practice setting: men and women 80 years and older, falls reduced by 30% |

     **Evidence-Based Falls Prevention, Second Edition**

| FIGURE 4.1 | Effective exercise programs tested in randomized controlled trials (cont.) |
|---|---|

| Article, sample | Exercise intervention | Evidence of effectiveness |
|---|---|---|
| Life Enrichment Activity Program (LEAP)<br><br>Keren Brown Wilson<br><br>Assisted Living Concepts, Inc.<br><br>Women aged 48–98, median age 81.6 in control, 84.2 in experimental group | • Fall prevention exercises, primarily active range of motion, for 30–45 minutes/day<br>• Residents advanced to beginning, intermediate, and advanced exercises as abilities improved<br>• Six-month program | • Falls increased in control group by 26%, decreased in exercise group by 26%<br>• Injuries related to falls decreased in control group by 33%, decreased in exercise group by 3.2%. |

## Sensory loss

Sensory loss is responsible for many preventable falls. Consider the following interventions for patients who are at risk of falling:

- A current eyeglass prescription is essential. In long-term care settings, every patient should have an ophthalmologist visit to identify and treat visual changes. In an acute-care setting, patients should be screened to identify new and recent sensory changes. If issues are identified, appropriate steps can be taken during their stay to assist them and prevent falls. In addition, consultations and referrals for post-discharge would be recommended to assist patients when they arrive home or to another level of patient care.

- Keep eyeglasses clean. Dirty or fogged eyeglasses may seriously impair vision and cause a fall.

- Single-vision eyeglasses are best. Bifocal, trifocal, and varifocal lenses can create moments of blurred vision, disorientation, and dizziness. Multifocal lenses frequently impair both depth perception and acuity. Patients are better off wearing glasses meant for normal distance viewing most of the time. Reading glasses should stay in a pocket or purse until needed.

- Hearing is a factor in balance and proprioception. Proprioception is the ability to sense the position, location, orientation, and movement of the body and its parts. It is a "sixth sense" that uses sensory receptors in the muscles, joints, and skin, as well as information from the eyes and ears, to send messages through the central nervous system that tell the body how to react to external forces and help us know when to move in response to something in our environment. Position in space is partly sensed by sound, so someone with impaired hearing may also have impaired balance. Encourage the use of hearing aids whenever a hearing-impaired patient is up and moving around, even in his or her own room.

- Eyeglasses and hearing aids must either be on the person or easily accessible to the person at all times.

Earwax obstructing the ear canal decreases hearing and impairs balance. Symptoms of impacted earwax include:

- Disturbance in balance
- Pain
- Tinnitus
- Nystagmus
- Nausea
- Cough

To prevent earwax accumulation, consider the following:

- Do not use cotton-tipped swabs or any other mechanical instrument to clean earwax.

- People with a tendency to accumulate earwax might benefit from regular ear drops.

- Try putting mineral, baby, or olive oil into the ears before bathing. Anything containing alcohol, bath soap, and shampoo may all cause earwax to harden. Water from washing may cause swelling of earwax and increase symptoms. Oil in the ears provides an earwax-softening barrier to these elements.

- Ear candles are not recommended and may cause injury.

**Evidence-Based Falls Prevention, Second Edition**

- Refer the patient to an ear, nose, and throat specialist for cleaning the earwax if the patient has pain, dizziness, inflammation, changes in hearing, or other suspected complications.[6]

Only a physician or someone trained, delegated, and supervised by a physician should attempt removal of earwax from the inner ear.

## Medication modifications

At a minimum, a review of every patient's medications with an eye toward fall reduction is essential. Nurses and pharmacists should ensure audits of the patients' medication regimens so that every patient's medications have been examined. When auditing, look for psychotropic medications, medications listed on Beers' criteria, diuretics that might cause toileting problems, and anyone taking more than four medications routinely. Consider the possibilities of alternative drugs or nonpharmacological treatments that might reduce the number of medications or the amount of medications with troubling side effects. Share your findings with the patients' physicians and encourage trial therapy to see whether other treatments might be just as successful with fewer falls.

In one study, intervention involved withdrawing participants from psychotropic medications gradually over a period of 14 weeks. Falls were reduced by 66% after 44 weeks, although the trial experienced a high dropout rate.[7]

## Psychological and cognitive modifications

Educating cognitively healthy patients and their families is an excellent intervention to combat some behavioral barriers. By providing patients and their families with as much knowledge as possible, they have some control over this aspect of their lives. When teaching, stress the value of fall prevention as a way to avoid serious injury and deterioration.

Patients' perceptions of their balance efficacy strongly influence their ability to move safely and respond effectively to loss of balance. People who are afraid of falling, either because they have fallen before or because they feel unsteady or weak, are more likely to fall. Exercise is one way to gradually combat this fear.

Although attempts have been made to combat fear of falling and reduce fall risk, research shows mixed results. It appears the multifaceted approaches that use both psychological and physical interventions may be the most successful to date.

If a patient shows a significant fear of falling, consider cognitive-behavioral interventions, along with education, exercise, and relaxation training. Improving the individual's confidence and self-efficacy may reduce the fear of falling and improve the ability to perform some of the functions of daily living.

The interventions that prevent falling in the cognitively normal are not always as successful for patients who have dementia. Falling is an inevitable part of the disease process in degenerative dementia disorders such as Alzheimer's disease. People with dementia will fall. However, some successes exist.

The current recommendation for preventing falls in the cognitively impaired is to take a practical approach, making many of the same modifications required for those without cognitive impairment:

- Even those patients with quite severe dementia are often able to cooperate to a surprising degree with interventions. Never assume that a patient can't comply with a modification just because he or she is cognitively impaired.

- Consider a broad range of fall causes. The patient may not be able to give a reliable history, and witnesses to falls may be unavailable. In the absence of hard facts, it is important to think about all the possible causes.

- Stopping medication is often worthwhile and not as difficult as many think.
    - Psychotropics prescribed during an acute episode may no longer be needed.
    - Since blood pressure often goes down as dementia worsens, hypotension becomes an issue. Review the need for previously prescribed antihypertensives.
    - A patient with angina who has become less mobile might not need previously prescribed antianginals.

- Assess cognitively impaired patients to determine the direction in which they are most likely to fall and the body parts they are most likely to injure. Patients with degenerative dementias tend to develop distinctive fall patterns, depending on the areas of the brain that are damaged and on muscular responses particular to the individual. Use padded clothing to protect body parts likely to be injured.

- Wearing soft, flexible moccasins or socks without shoes enables the cognitively impaired patient to feel the floor and compensate for declining proprioception, reducing falls.

- OH is easily diagnosed and potentially treatable. Consider assessing it with continuous monitoring equipment, such as the noninvasive blood pressure monitor that continuously measures arterial blood pressure in the finger. This type of assessment is well tolerated and accurate.

- Some people with dementia can be helped by physical therapy.

- Small interventions can make big improvements in mobility. Changing a walking aid to something more appropriate or wearing suitable shoes may make a big difference.

- Hip protectors (soft padded clothing-type protectors are the most easily tolerated by patients with dementia), knee pads, elbow pads, wrist splints, and soft foam helmets have shown great efficacy in reducing or eliminating serious injuries in people who fall.

- Medication/supplementation with vitamin D and calcium to prevent fractures may be indicated for dementia sufferers with osteoporosis.

Dementia sufferers lose visual acuity and the ability to recognize three-dimensional objects. The world of someone with cognitive impairment can be similar to the distorted images of a fun-house mirror—nothing looks like it used to, with some images blending into others and some things becoming smaller, larger, or differently shaped. For a patient with dementia, multidimensional objects sometimes appear to flatten out against the surrounding environment. Imagine a woman with beginning stage dementia related to alcoholism sitting down to eat at a table covered with a white tablecloth and set with a white plate and silverware. The scene may make no sense to her at all, because all she sees is a field of white with nothing to distinguish the objects on the table. Many times, someone with cognitive impairment won't eat simply because he or she doesn't recognize the utensils. This same loss of perceptual understanding contributes to fall risk, because in the absence of sharply distinguishing characteristics or colors, many objects in a dementia sufferer's visual field flatten out and merge with the background. As a result, patients with dementia may trip over things they don't recognize as having solid dimensions.

Another frequent result of cognitive impairment is loss of judgment. This is particularly difficult because the sufferer usually doesn't realize his or her judgment is impaired. Someone with dementia might fearlessly wander across a highway with no regard for the speeding cars, because he or she can no longer connect actions with consequences. Or the cognitively impaired patient might believe that a dark carpet is actually a large hole that he or she will fall into, so he or she refuses to walk into a room.

It is often hard to know what motivates the dementia sufferer's seemingly irrational actions; however, the behavior we see is always purposeful and motivated by reasons that make sense to the individual. Because the cognitively impaired person is operating in a world based on distorted perceptions and thought processes, he or she is bound to collide with the physical world in one way or another, often with a fall.

## Environmental modifications

The first step in reducing environmental causes of falls in a hospital is to educate every staff member about them. Environmental falls are accidents waiting to happen. Accidents may not be predictable but they are preventable with attention to environmental risk factors. The first thing staff should know is that it is their responsibility to prevent falls, especially those due to environmental factors that could be removed. Figure 4.2 lists considerations that all staff should bear in mind.

| FIGURE 4.2 | Daily staff considerations for fall prevention |
|---|---|

- The first person who sees an object where it doesn't belong (e.g., on the floor, blocking a pathway) is responsible for picking it up or moving it—immediately.

- The first person who sees a wet or slick spot on the floor or ground is responsible for cleaning it up—immediately.

- Anyone who sees a rough piece of flooring, such as wrinkled carpet, is responsible for fixing it or getting it fixed—immediately.

- Anyone who sees a light bulb that is out or a light fixture that isn't working is responsible for getting a new light bulb or finding someone who can fix the problem as soon as possible.

- Cords or hoses trailing across pathways must be pulled up, or the pathway must be marked and blocked while the equipment is being used. Staff should be alert for trailing electrical cords in patients' rooms.

- Anyone who notices that a patient's eyeglasses are dirty or that the patient is wearing pants that are too long or heels that are too high is responsible for helping the patient clean the eyeglasses and put on appropriate clothes.

It only takes a second for a hazard to become the cause of a serious fall. No environmental risk factor should be allowed to remain in place any longer than the time it takes someone to notice it.

## Medical interventions

In addition to conscientious management of chronic diseases such as Parkinson's and multiple sclerosis, some specific medical conditions are responsible for a number of falls and often are overlooked.

Orthostatic hypotension (OH) is a reduction of systolic blood pressure of at least 20 mmHg, a reduction of diastolic blood pressure of at least 10 mmHg, or a drop in systolic blood pressure to 90 mmHg or less within three minutes of standing. It has been observed in all age groups, but, like dementia, occurs more frequently in the elderly. There are many different causes for OH, a few of which are summarized in Figure 4.3.

**FIGURE 4.3** — **Frequent causes of OH**

Low intravascular volume:
- Inadequate fluid intake
- Diarrhea
- Hemorrhage
- Adrenal insufficiency
- Diabetes insipidus
- Dehydration
- Burns
- Vomiting
- Salt-losing nephropathy

Medications:
- Antihypertensives (diuretics, beta blockers, calcium-channel blockers, ACE inhibitors)
- Antiparkinsonian (levodopa, bromocriptine, selegiline)
- Antidepressants (tricyclics, SSRIs, trazodone)
- Antipsychotics (clozapine, haloperidol)
- Nitrates
- Minor tranquilizers
- Insulin

Immobility:
Parkinson's disease, multiple sclerosis, diabetes mellitus, renal failure, brain tumors, pure autonomic failure, brain-stem lesions, carotid sinus hypersensitivity

Any patient who has had a fall or an episode of syncope should be evaluated for OH. Symptoms may include lightheadedness, dizziness, blurred vision, fatigue, weakness, nausea, palpitations, tremulousness, headache, neck pain, and cognitive impairment. Sometimes people experience OH with no symptoms at all. The condition can occur intermittently, varying with the time of day, food intake, and medication use. OH is most prevalent first thing in the morning.

Repeated blood pressure measurements may be required to confirm a clinical finding of OH. Individuals should be supine for at least five minutes (10 minutes is preferable) before having their blood pressure and heart rate taken to ensure a stable reading. Then their blood pressure and heart rate should be measured when they first stand up and again three minutes later. Simply taking the blood pressure reading when the individual sits and then stands is not sufficient for diagnosing OH. If the systolic blood pressure drops at least 20 mmHg or the diastolic by at least 10 mmHg within three minutes of standing from a supine position, a clinical finding of OH is reasonable. Morning measurements are more reproducible, and continuous monitoring is even more likely to make a diagnosis of OH.

The interventions for OH depend on its cause. For example, low fluid volume caused by inadequate fluid intake is treated by increasing fluid intake and adding liberal salt to the diet, unless contraindicated. Address other causes of low intravascular volume by finding hemorrhage and stopping it or by treating diarrhea. Medications that can cause OH should be examined, and their clinical benefit should be weighed against their adverse effects. Unnecessary medications should be discontinued, and necessary drugs should have their dosage interval increased or their doses decreased, if this can be done while still achieving the desired therapeutic benefit. A physician should examine an individual with OH to look for possible underlying causes such as anemia, autonomic failure, and secondary autonomic disorders.

Exercise can make OH worse by causing skeletal muscle vasodilation. Prolonged inactivity, however, also worsens OH. Exercise in a horizontal position, such as during swimming, can be beneficial. On the whole, exercise should be encouraged, though staff must keep in mind that some types of exercise could exacerbate OH.

People with OH should be advised to change body positions slowly to allow their body time to adapt, especially in the morning and after meals. They should stay well hydrated and avoid alcohol. Elevating the head of the bed to 30 degrees by using wooden blocks has been found to reduce OH. In one study, leg-crossing and squatting improved OH by increasing blood pressure in people with autonomic dysfunction.[8] Compression stockings that go to the waist may be helpful, but they are difficult to put on and take off, hot, and contraindicated in people with skin ulcers. Nonpharmacological treatments for OH are summarized in Figure 4.4.

| FIGURE 4.4 | Nonpharmacological treatments for OH |
|---|---|

| Measures to be avoided | Measures to be tried |
|---|---|
| Sudden head-up postural changes | Head tilted up during sleep |
| Lying down for prolonged periods | High salt intake |
| Warm environments | Crossing legs, squatting, bending forward, physical maneuvers with legs |
| Alcohol | Thigh-high or waist-high compression stockings if not contraindicated and/or abdominal binders |
| Large meals, especially those heavy with carbohydrates, particularly simple sugars | Small, frequent meals with limited simple sugars |
| Straining during defecation or micturition | Exercise, especially swimming |
| Medications with hypotensive side effects | Caffeine with meals |

Postprandial hypotension (PPH) is distinct from OH but may occur in conjunction with it. PPH is defined as a decrease in systolic blood pressure of 20 mmHg or more within two hours of the start of a meal. PPH may be even more common than OH. Large, carbohydrate-rich meals increase the magnitude of the blood pressure drop in those with this syndrome. Simple carbohydrates, such as sugar, frequently produce this problem. Coffee or some other caffeinated beverage at the end of a meal may be helpful in preventing the drop in blood pressure.

## Cardiovascular causes of falls

Cardiovascular disorders are common causes of falls. These disorders are dangerous but treatable, either with a pacemaker or medications, which makes it imperative to give careful consideration to these disorders when assessing patients with unexplained or recurrent falls. If a patient falls without attempting to stop the fall or self-rescue, consider a cardiovascular cause and request a cardiovascular workup.

# References

1. Bischoff, H. A., and Brigham, R. B. (2003). "The importance of maximizing vitamin D in the elderly diet with respect to function and falls." *Geriatrics & Aging* 6:(7): 41–44.

2. Ibid.

3. Buchner, D., Cress M., De Lateur, B, et al. (1997). "The effect of strength and endurance training on gait, balance, fall risk, and health services use in community-living older adults." *J Gerontol A (Biol Sci Med Sci)* 52: M218–224.

4. Campbell, A., Robertson, C., Gardner, M., Norton R., and Buchner, D. (1999). "Falls prevention over 2 years: A randomized controlled trial in women 80 years and older." *Age Ageing*; 28: 513–1518.

5. Robertson, M.C., Devlin, N., Gardner, M., Campbell, J. "Effectiveness and economic evaluation of a nurse delivered home exercise programme to prevent falls: A randomised controlled trial." *Br Med J 2001*; 322: 697–701.

6. Carne, S. (1980). "Ear syringing." *British Medical Journal*; 280:374.

7. Brymer, C. (2000)."Going from research to practice: Three falls prevention trials." *Geriatrics & Aging*; 3:(6):13. *www.geriatricsandaging.com*.

8. Grant, M. (2003)."Treatment of orthostatic hypotension: Preserving function and quality of life." *Geriatrics & Aging* 6:7. *www.geriatricsandaging.com*.

# CHAPTER 5:

## Fall-prevention programs

## Learning objectives

After reading this chapter, the participant should be able to:

- Identify hospitalwide steps that may reduce the risk of falls
- List modifiable risk factors that a good fall-prevention program should address
- Identify the three main elements of a fall-prevention program
- Identify elements that should be included in a multifactorial intervention program

## Introduction

Every individual and agency that cares for people has a different fall risk profile. The first thing to remember about developing a fall-prevention program is that fall prevention interventions must be individualized to each patient and each hospital. No two people fall for exactly the same reason, and no prescribed set of interventions will work for everyone.

Designing patient-specific interventions is the most important part of any fall-prevention program. Generic, one-size-fits-all programs usually don't fit any one patient very well and have limited usefulness. Although we must teach all staff members the general safety precautions that apply in every situation, such as cleaning up spills and eliminating clutter, these are in no way sufficient to significantly reduce falls in any hospital. Unless targeted interventions are planned for each patient, a fall-prevention program is doomed for failure.

Some hospitalwide steps exist that may reduce the risk of falls. Facilities should incorporate the following:

• Staff education programs to raise awareness of fall risk and teach prevention measures. The information in this manual could provide several hours of education.

• Regular review of every patient's medications, particularly psychotropics.

• Regular review of each patient's fall history and the hospital/unit annual fall statistics.

• Balance and gait screenings of all patients.
  - A simple balance and gait screening is the "Get Up and Go" test. Ask the patient to stand up from a seated position in a straight-backed chair without using his or her arms, walk several paces, and return to the chair. Time how long this activity takes. A common approach to this is the "Eight-Foot Get Up and Go" test, where the patient walks around a cone eight feet away from the chair and then returns to a sitting position. Walking assistance devices are allowed if they are normally used. The patient should be told to walk at a speed that is comfortable to him or her, wearing normal footwear. Less than 20 seconds is an acceptable time. Anything slower than 30 seconds indicates a problem.

  - Refer anyone who has difficulty with this test for further assessment and appropriate intervention, such as a physical therapy or occupational therapy consultation. Those who take from 20 to 29 seconds could probably benefit from therapy and should be evaluated. This test is considered the single best assessment for geriatric patients who experience a fall.

• Review of staffing patterns in light of the pattern of falls in the hospital. Ask:
  - When do most of our falls occur?
  - How many staff members are normally on duty during those times?
  - Is there a correlation between the incidence of falls and the number of staff on duty?
  - Can we make adjustments to staffing patterns to accommodate high fall-risk times?

     **Evidence-Based Falls Prevention, Second Edition**

• Patient and family education programs. Several good videos are available for teaching patients and families about fall risk and prevention. Presenting portions of this manual would be helpful as well. The more patients and families know and understand about this problem, the more support they will be able to give the facility in preventing falls, and the less likely they will be to blame the facility for a fall when they know that everything possible is being done to prevent them.

Multifaceted programs that include assessment of environmental, medical, functional, and psychological risk factors, health professionals' advice, and provision of risk-modifying interventions have been shown to work in acute-care settings with extensive staff training and support by professional specialists. We can modify most risk factors by proactive identification and intervention.

The FICSIT trial studies show that intervening in the following risk factors demonstrates a reduction in falls:[1]

• Orthostatic hypotension (OH)
• Sedative/hypnotic medications
• Use of more than four medications
• Toilet and bath safety
• Environmental hazards
• Abnormal gait, transfers, and balance
• Lower and upper extremity strength and range of motion
• Foot problems

All of these risk factors are modifiable. A good fall-prevention program will address each of these eight factors through programs such as medication review, safety committee audits, incident investigations, exercise programs, and careful assessment of individual patients.

## Developing a fall-prevention program

There are three main elements to a fall-prevention program. The first is assessing the patients to identify the risk factors facing each individual and the hospital as a whole. The second is planning interventions to address the risk factors. The third is modifying the risk factors, partly through extensive staff, patient, and family education.

### *Patient assessment and risk factor identification*

Every patient admitted to a hospital should be assessed for fall risk upon admission. Every time a patient falls, assess the patient again for fall risk. This assessment can be undertaken in a variety of ways, using a number of available tools. Figure 5.1 examines elements that must be addressed during these assessments.

Patients who are at risk for falling may need to be identified in some way, depending on your hospital's policies. For instance, patients with high fall risks could be identified with "falling" stars or leaves. Place the falling stars on patient's medical records, on their doors, or in their rooms to alert staff to the patient's particular fall risk issues. Be conscious of the Health Insurance Portability and Accountability Act of 1996's (HIPAA's) regulations and privacy concerns if you use this kind of identification system.

Also consider implementing a stoplight system, which involves posting a picture of a stoplight in a patient's room with either a red, yellow, or green light, with these meanings:

- A red light means the patient should not be up without assistance and cannot be left unattended when in the bathroom.
- A yellow light means the patient requires a minimum of standby assistance for any activity.
- A green light means the patient may be up without assistance.

Figures 5.2 and 5.3 feature fall assessment tools that can be used to monitor patients. At best, risk assessment can identify that a patient has a potential to fall. It cannot tell you why the patient is at risk of falling or how to intervene. Risk assessment highlights for the caregiver that there is a need to further assess and determine the best interventions for the specific person.

    **Evidence-Based Falls Prevention, Second Edition**

**FIGURE 5.1**                    Fall assessment guidelines

**Inquire about fall history:**
- For those with one or more recent falls or those reporting recurrent falls, obtain history of fall circumstances. If there was a loss of consciousness or no memory of the fall(s), inquire about witnesses.

**Inquire about fall risk factors:**
- Medications, prescribed and over-the-counter
- Acute and chronic medical problems (including alcoholism)
- Mobility levels

**Physical assessment:**
- Anyone who reports a history of a single fall should undergo balance and gait screening. Observe the individual's ability to stand up from a chair without using his or her arms, walk several paces, and return. This is known as the "get up and go" test.

- Anyone who has difficulty with the "get up and go" test should undergo further assessment and intervention, such as physical or occupational therapy.

- Examine/assess:
  ✓ Vision (contrast sensitivity and peripheral vision)
  ✓ Muscle strength and tone
  ✓ Gait
  ✓ Balance
  ✓ Lower-extremity function
  ✓ Feet and shoes
  ✓ Neurological function:
    - Lower-extremity peripheral nerves
    - proprioception
    - reflexes
  ✓ Cognitive function
  ✓ Cardiovascular evaluation:
    - heart rate and rhythm
    - orthostatic pulse
    - orthostatic blood pressure (sitting, standing, lying)
  ✓ Toileting needs:
    - urinalysis to detect urinary-tract infections
    - diuretics causing nighttime toileting

**FIGURE 5.1**  **Fall assessment guidelines (cont.)**

✓ lab values:
- red blood-cell count
- white blood-cell count
- blood glucose
- medication levels (Dilantin, Lanoxin, others that might be toxic)
  ✓ weight changes
  ✓ medication changes
  ✓ alcohol use

**Physical therapists' considerations:**

- Range of motion
- Flexibility
- Strength
- Gait

- Balance
- Assistive devices
- Footwear
- E-stimulation

- Soft tissue techniques
- Pain management
- Ultrasound

**Occupational therapists' considerations:**

- Fine motor coordination
- Eye-hand coordination
- Range of motion
- Flexibility

- Energy conservation
- Low-vision techniques
- Posture
- Cognitive tasks

- Strength
- Environmental adaptations
- Safety awareness

**Speech therapists' considerations:**

- Competency
- Attention deficit

- Cognition
- Safety awareness

| FIGURE 5.2 | Sample Morse risk assessment tool |
|---|---|

This tool, designed for use in an acutecare setting, has been rigorously tested for statistical reliability and validity. Each category of risk carries a particular weight. The risk categories are history of falls, secondary diagnosis, mobility aids, attachment to equipment, gait, and mental status. When assessing someone with this tool, use the criteria in each category to assign an individual score for that particular risk. After scoring every category, add the scores. The total score, which can be anywhere from zero to 125, indicates the individual's level of risk. A score of 45 or greater indicates a high fall risk.

| Item | | | Score |
|---|---|---|---|
| History of falling | No = 0 | Yes = 25 <br> A fall immediately prior to admission, fall during present admission, or one fall every six months in long-term care. | |
| Secondary diagnosis | No = 0 | Yes = 15 <br> Two or more medical diagnoses are listed on the patient's chart. | |
| Walking aid | None/bed rest/wheelchair/nurse assist = 0 <br> Walks independently or is assisted, or uses a wheelchair safely or is on bed rest and does not get out of bed at all without total assistance. | Crutches/cane/walker = 15 <br><br> Furniture = 30 <br> Walks clutching furniture for support. | |
| IV therapy/ pump | No = 0 | Yes = 20 <br> IV, heparin or saline lock | |
| Gait | Normal/bed rest/wheelchair/immobile = 10 <br> Patient has normal gait, head is erect, arms swinging freely, or is on bed rest or immobile. | Weak = 20 <br> Patient has a weak gait with stooped posture or uses the support of furniture with featherweight touch. Steps are short or may shuffle. <br><br> Impaired = 20 <br> Patient has difficulty rising from chair, is poor balance, grasps on to furniture or a support person, or uses a walking aid for support, or cannot walk without assistance. | |
| Mental status | Oriented to own ability = 0 <br> Patient's self-assessment of own ability matches nurse's/physician's assessment or orders. | Overestimates/forgets limitations = 15 <br> Patient is unrealistic or overestimates his or her abilities and is forgetful of limitations. | |
| | | Total Score | |
| | Score > 0 = Provide universal fall precautions | | |
| | Score > 45 = Initiate falls protocol, initiate or revise falls plan of care | A score of 45 or greater means the patient is at high risk for falls. | |
| | Score > 75 = Consult falls nurse | | |

Source: Morse, J.M. (2002). "Enhancing the safety of hospitalization by reducing patient falls." American Journal of Infection Control. 30:(6):376–380.

**FIGURE 5.3**     **Fall risk evaluation tool**

Check each of the following criteria that apply to the patient being assessed. A patient who shows the presence of any of the criteria in the general category/more than one of the other categories (physical status, mental status, medication, ambulatory device, or other) should be considered at risk for falling.

General data category

_____ History of previous falls

_____ Functional-assessment score > 50, with a mental status questionnaire score < 23

Physical status category     _____ Fatigability     _____ Sight impairment

_____ Dizziness/balance problems   _____ Debilitated or weak     _____ Hearing impairment

_____ Unsteady gait     _____ Paresis     _____ History of alcoholism

_____ Joint difficulties     _____ Seizure disorder

Mental status category

_____ Confusion (illogical thinking)     _____ Lack of familiarity with immediate surroundings

_____ Impaired memory and judgment     _____ Inability to understand/follow directions

_____ Disoriented to person/place/time     _____ Nocturnal disorientation

Medication category

_____ Drugs that have a diuretic effect

_____ Drugs that suppress thought processes/create a hypotensive effect (e.g., narcotics, sedatives, psychotropics, hypnotics, tranquilizers, antidepressive drugs, and antihypertensives)

_____ Drugs that increase gastrointestinal motility (i.e., laxatives, enemas, and cathartics)

Ambulatory device category

_____ Walker     _____ Wheelchair

_____ Crutches     _____ Gerichair

_____ Cane

Restraining device category

_____ Jacket restraint     _____ Soft restraint

_____ Belt restraint     _____ Gerichair tabletop

_____ Vest restraint     _____ Side rails

     **Evidence-Based Falls Prevention, Second Edition**

| FIGURE 5.3 | Fall risk evaluation tool (cont.) |

Other category

_____ Emotional upsets or loss of significant person

_____ A recent escape from restraints

_____ History of crawling out of bed

_____ Unwillingness to call for help with walking

_____ Improperly fitting footwear

Implementation

1. The final decision as to whether a patient is at risk to fall is based on your nursing judgment. If patient is assessed as being at high risk for falls:

a. Initiate a system for identifying this individual's high risk for falls so all staff will be aware.

b. Initiate the individualized nursing care plan based on the nursing diagnosis potential for injury.

c. The patient is (check one):

_____ At a high risk to fall

_____ Not at a high risk to fall.

Nurse's signature _____

Date _____

Adapted from: Young, S.W., Abedzadeh, C.B., and White, M.W. (1989). "A fall-prevention program for nursing homes." *Nursing Management* 20:80Y-80AA, 80DD, 80FF.

## Intervention planning

As we noted previously, the most successful intervention programs are multifactorial, addressing multiple possible causes and risk factors. Successful interventions are also individualized, developed for each patient based on a careful assessment of that individual's condition and situation. Interventions that include a detailed medical assessment followed by referral to appropriate services, such as ophthalmologists and therapists, consistently result in a reduction in fall risk.

Multifactorial intervention programs should include these elements:

- Gait/transfer training by physical therapists.

- Assistive device training and fitting by physical therapists.

- Obtaining and teaching use of assistive devices by occupational therapists.

- Individualized exercise programs including:
    - Balance training
    - Lower- and upper-extremity strength
    - Lower- and upper-extremity range of motion

- Review and modification of medication regimens, especially psychotropic and sympath-omimetic drugs. Reduce overall medications taken when possible.

- Treatment of postural hypotension.

- Treatment of cardiovascular disorders, including carotid sinus syndrome and arrhythmias.

- Modification of environmental hazards, including toilet and bath safety, with appropriate adaptive devices, bath mats, and assistance.

- Treatment of foot problems.

- Appropriate footwear and clothing.

- Addressing sensory deficits with vision and hearing evaluation and correction/aids.

Interventions should always be planned to address the problems identified in the assessment. Interventions that are appropriate for a patient are incorporated into the patient's care plan.

Once you have assessed a patient and planned specific interventions, implement the interventions and have a system for evaluating their effectiveness. The first step requires thorough education of staff, patients, and family members.

# Educating staff, patients, and family members

Use the resources in this manual to help plan training sessions. Teach the risk factors that are responsible for falls and the specific modifications that can prevent falls. Help staff, patients, and family members understand the root causes of falls so they can appreciate the importance of the interventions you want to implement.

Basic environmental interventions apply to everyone in a hospital and to the hospital as a whole. Stress to staff that fall prevention is everyone's responsibility. Plan and conduct repeated training sessions for staff, patients, and families. Enlist the assistance of nurses, physical therapists, and occupational therapists for these sessions. The primary goal is to teach prevention, but this is also a good time to teach the patients and families how to respond to a fall when it occurs. Demonstrate how to gently assist patients to the ground if they have lost their balance. Teach patients how to have a "good fall," by showing self-rescue techniques such as backing up against a wall and sliding down it.

You need a system in place for implementing patient-specific interventions. Putting the interventions on the patient's care plan is the first step. Emphasize these interventions at every care meeting. Holding the staff accountable for implementing the interventions is essential. This accountability can be provided through routine follow-up and evaluation of the success of the interventions.

# Track and trend systems

Accountability requires a way to track and trend falls that occur in your hospital. Examine each patient's history of falls and evaluate interventions in place. Ask these questions:

- Is the patient complying with the interventions? If not, why?
- Is the staff implementing the interventions? If not, why?
- Are the interventions effective? (The measure of effectiveness is whether the number of falls has been reduced.)
- If the interventions aren't effective, what different interventions should be tried?

Every fall should lead to a reassessment of the patient in question, taking a close look at the cause of the fall and the interventions that were implemented. Every fall requires an incident report, which should be the starting point of the investigation into why the fall occurred and what needs to be done to prevent further falls. Figure 5.4 outlines a "decision tree" that staff can use to decide what to do when a fall occurs.

 **Evidence-Based Falls Prevention, Second Edition**

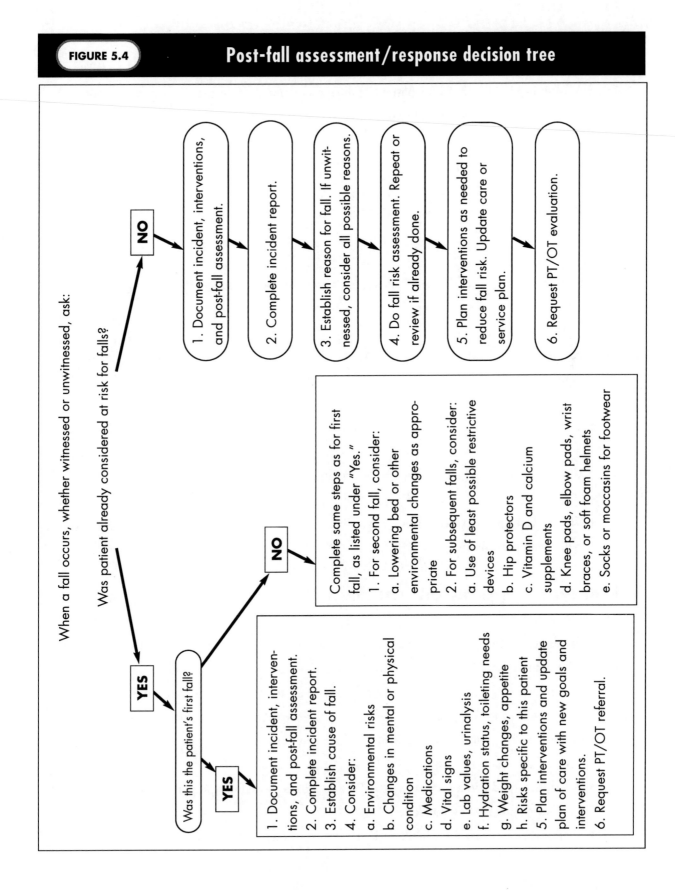

**FIGURE 5.4**

Post-fall assessment/response decision tree

When a fall occurs, whether witnessed or unwitnessed, ask:

Was patient already considered at risk for falls?

**NO**

1. Document incident, interventions, and post-fall assessment.

2. Complete incident report.

3. Establish reason for fall. If unwitnessed, consider all possible reasons.

4. Do fall risk assessment. Repeat or review if already done.

5. Plan interventions as needed to reduce fall risk. Update care or service plan.

6. Request PT/OT evaluation.

**YES**

Was this the patient's first fall?

**NO**

Complete same steps as for first fall, as listed under "Yes."

1. For second fall, consider:
   a. Lowering bed or other environmental changes as appropriate

2. For subsequent falls, consider:
   a. Use of least possible restrictive devices
   b. Hip protectors
   c. Vitamin D and calcium supplements
   d. Knee pads, elbow pads, wrist braces, or soft foam helmets
   e. Socks or moccasins for footwear

**YES**

1. Document incident, interventions, and post-fall assessment.

2. Complete incident report.

3. Establish cause of fall.

4. Consider:
   a. Environmental risks
   b. Changes in mental or physical condition
   c. Medications
   d. Vital signs
   e. Lab values, urinalysis
   f. Hydration status, toileting needs
   g. Weight changes, appetite
   h. Risks specific to this patient

5. Plan interventions and update plan of care with new goals and interventions.

6. Request PT/OT referral.

# Sample hospitalwide fall-prevention programs

Every so often, examine all of your patients' fall risk assessments together. Do you have a high fall-risk hospital? If so, there are a number of things to consider. Ask these questions:

- Why are people falling?

- What staffing patterns might need adjustment to accommodate times when falls tend to occur?

- How can you program patients' activities to provide optimal supervision during times when falls are likely to occur?

- How can you provide rest periods for those who are easily fatigued, such as patients with dementia? Many falls occur toward the end of the day, when patients are tired.

- What environmental hazards do you need to address?

- What programs can you implement that will provide opportunities for safe movement?

- What educational opportunities can you provide staff, patients, and family members that will help them prevent falls?

# Fall-prevention program checkup

A regular assessment of your fall-prevention program should involve a review of falls by your safety committee, which should include representatives from administration, the kitchen, maintenance, housekeeping, nursing, and direct caregivers. Examine all the patient falls that have occurred since the last review. During safety committee meetings, ask the following questions to determine the root cause of the incident, remembering that more than one of the items may be a contributing factor:

- **Procedures and patient assessment:** Were adequate procedures/proper patient assessment(s) in place to prevent the incident?
- **Training/awareness:** Were staff, patient(s)/guest(s) aware of applicable procedures?

- **Procedures followed:** Were hospital fall-prevention procedures/rules followed?
- **Equipment:** Did staff/patients use the proper equipment in the right way?
- **Communication:** Did proper communication occur between staff and patient(s)?

Prior to each meeting, safety committee members should take turns conducting a walk-through safety audit of the hospital. Discuss each deficiency in the audit with the committee. Discuss staff training needs and ask each attendee whether they have any safety concerns they want the committee to address. The concerns should include any physical hazards they have observed or care issues for a patient that may cause an injury.

An important function of a safety committee is to analyze incident reports and determine the root cause of each incident. The root cause is the underlying reason that something occurred. For example, if a patient slipped and fell in the hallway, what really caused the fall? Was the cause something intrinsic, a condition specific to the patient such as postural hypotension or carotid sinus syndrome? Or was it extrinsic, due to a torn piece of carpet or shoes with thick, rubbery soles that caught on the carpet pile? It should be the committee's responsibility to get to the bottom of each incident in the facility. Once the root cause is determined, an intervention plan should be developed to fix the problem. In the case of falling incidents, there are often several root causes, all of which must be addressed in a multifactorial intervention plan.

## Falls documentation

Document the root-cause analyses of events in a format similar to the one outlined in Figure 5.5. Document identified fall hazards that require staff follow-up using a chart similar to Figure 5.6.

Record each fall in a tracking document that shows all the falls occurring in the hospital over a specified period of time, usually a month or a quarter (see Figure 5.7). Record the cause of the fall and the outcome. Watch these records closely and look for trends, such as an increase in "slip and falls," which might indicate the need for staff education. Do an analysis of the trends at least quarterly to consider what hospitalwide interventions you might need to implement.

Another hospitalwide initiative that could take place includes the use of a falls unit audit. These audits can be completed on patients who have been on the unit for at least one complete shift. Figure 5.8 is a standard form for a falls audit, provided by the University Hospital at UAB in Birmingham, AL.

| FIGURE 5.5 | Fall documentation and root-cause analysis |
|---|---|

| Date: | Description: |
|---|---|
| | Root cause(s): (e.g., environmental—cleanliness, physical factors, staffing factors) |
| | Recommendation/corrective action: |
| | Person assigned:<br>Projected completion date: |

| FIGURE 5.6 | Hazard identification documentation |
|---|---|

| Hazard identification/recommendation for correction | Person assigned | Projected completion date |
|---|---|---|
| | | |
| | | |
| | | |
| | | |
| | | |

   **Evidence-Based Falls Prevention, Second Edition**

| FIGURE 5.7 | | Fall-tracking document |

**Unadjusted Incidents by Month and Shift**

| Type of Fall | Shift | JAN | FEB | MAR | APR | MAY | JUN | JUL | AUG | SEP | OCT | NOV | DEC | Annual Total | Annual Average |
|---|---|---|---|---|---|---|---|---|---|---|---|---|---|---|---|
| Fall without injury | 7-3 | | | | | | | | | | | | | | |
| | 3-11 | | | | | | | | | | | | | | |
| | 11-7 | | | | | | | | | | | | | | |
| | Subtotal | | | | | | | | | | | | | | |
| Fall with minor injury | 7-3 | | | | | | | | | | | | | | |
| | 3-11 | | | | | | | | | | | | | | |
| | 11-7 | | | | | | | | | | | | | | |
| | Subtotal | | | | | | | | | | | | | | |
| Fall with major injury | 7-3 | | | | | | | | | | | | | | |
| | 3-11 | | | | | | | | | | | | | | |
| | 11-7 | | | | | | | | | | | | | | |
| | Subtotal | | | | | | | | | | | | | | |
| Total all falls for shift and month | 7-3 | | | | | | | | | | | | | | |
| | 3-11 | | | | | | | | | | | | | | |
| | 11-7 | | | | | | | | | | | | | | |
| | Total | | | | | | | | | | | | | | |
| Average per shift and month | 7-3 | | | | | | | | | | | | | | |
| | 3-11 | | | | | | | | | | | | | | |
| | 11-7 | | | | | | | | | | | | | | |
| | Avg. | | | | | | | | | | | | | | |
| Average # patients | | | | | | | | | | | | | | | |
| # days in month | | 31 | 28 | 31 | 30 | 31 | 30 | 31 | 31 | 30 | 31 | 30 | 31 | | |

**Adjusted falls per patients per 30 days**

| | JAN | FEB | MAR | APR | MAY | JUN | JUL | AUG | SEP | OCT | NOV | DEC | Annual Total | Annual Average |
|---|---|---|---|---|---|---|---|---|---|---|---|---|---|---|
| Falls without injury | | | | | | | | | | | | | | |
| Falls with minor injury | | | | | | | | | | | | | | |
| Falls with major injury | | | | | | | | | | | | | | |
| Month total | | | | | | | | | | | | | | |

**FIGURE 5.8**            Falls standard audit

Patient name: _____

MR #:_____

Unit:_____

Admitting diagnosis:_____

Auditor:_____

Admitting nurse:_____

Date of audit:_____

Nurse of shift:_____

1. Falls risk completed on admission?  Y  N
2. Is the patient at risk for falls? (If "yes," continue)  Y  N
3. Fall precautions indicated.  Y  N
4. Rail is up, and marked, if appropriate.  Y  N
5. Bed is in low position.  Y  N
6. Call light is in reach.  Y  N
7. Bed alarm is indicated.  Y  N
8. Fall identified as a problem on Problem List.  Y  N
9. Medic alert or nurse-to-nurse entry of fall risk.  Y  N
10. Patient education took place regarding falls.  Y  N
11. "Falling Star" is in place on the door.  Y  N
12. "Falling Star" is in place on patient board.  Y  N
13. "Falling Star" is in place on chart.  Y  N
14. Fall risk purple armband is on patient.  Y  N
15. Wheels are locked (bed, chair, or wheelchair).  Y  N

*Source: Melanie Schultz, MSN, CN, APRN, BC, and Terry Motes, RN, BSN, MPA, ONC, CNA-BC, University Hospital at UAB. Adapted with permission.*

# References

1. (1994). "Frailty and injuries cooperative studies of intervention techniques: A multifactorial intervention to reduce the risk of falling among elderly people living in the community." *New England Journal of Medicine* 331:821–827.

# CHAPTER 6:

## Fall response

# 6

# Fall response

## Learning objectives

After reading this chapter, the participant should be able to:

- Formulate questions to ask after a fall takes place in order to respond appropriately
- Describe factors to consider when conducting a post-fall assessment of an unwitnessed fall
- Identify three distinct information records that must be maintained for every fall

## Fall response

Rapid and appropriate response to a fall can be the difference between a correctable problem and a fatal one, for a variety of reasons:

- Only a brief time on the floor after a fall can lead to additional complications, such as shock and dehydration. Any delay in treatment is a potential danger to the patient.

- The first few minutes after any medical crisis are the most critical in determining the outcome, so if a fall has occurred as a result of a cardiac, circulatory, or neurological problem, immediate and appropriate care is required to prevent permanent damage or death.

- Even if the fall is minor, caused by a simple trip or slip, reacting immediately can prevent further injury to the patient who fell and to others who might be affected by any environmental hazards, including the hazard of an individual on the floor blocking a pathway.

- Fast response to a fall is necessary to help determine the cause of the fall, providing essential information to help prevent future falls.

- Quick arrival on the scene establishes crucial assessment data, such as level of consciousness, which will help determine the kind of treatment needed.

- The longer someone is on the floor without assistance, the more frightened they become, putting extreme stress on already compromised immune responses and organ systems.

- If help is not readily and immediately available, an individual's attempts to help him or herself may cause additional injury.

## Questions to ask

When someone falls, a number of things must be determined at once. Answers to some of these questions will make a difference in how we should respond:

### Why did the patient fall?

If the person fell because of a cardiac or neurological problem, such as a heart attack, blood pressure drop, or stroke, injuries from the fall may be the least of our concerns. It is more important to recognize that a medical problem has occurred and respond appropriately. Any time a patient falls and is unconscious or cannot say what caused the fall, consider cardiac, circulatory, or neurological disorders as potential causes. Any of these might require immediate medical care to prevent further damage from occurring to the brain or heart. This kind of fall requires an emergency response, since death or permanent disability might result without rapid intervention.

If the patient fell because of an environmental hazard, the most urgent concern is removing the person from further danger and examining the scene to prevent more falls. A quick survey of the environment might reveal water on the floor or something else in the area that caused the fall.

 **Evidence-Based Falls Prevention, Second Edition**

### What injuries have occurred?

Falls are responsible for many fatal brain injuries. Even a seemingly minor bump on the head can cause dangerous bruising or bleeding in the brain. Find out whether the patient lost consciousness, even for a moment, either before or after the fall.

Loss of consciousness before a fall indicates a medical condition that must be investigated. Loss of consciousness as a result of hitting the head during a fall indicates the possibility of severe brain injury, even if no signs of head trauma are visible. Symptoms of a serious head injury can be delayed, which is why patients should be monitored every two to three hours for at least 24 hours after any trauma to the head, as well as checked periodically thereafter for several days.

Knowing what injuries may have occurred dictates the response to the fall. The possibility of head and neck injuries and fractures should be assumed whenever a fall occurs. Unless the patient must be removed from danger, he or she should not be moved until a comprehensive assessment has been performed. Hip fractures, so common in the elderly, may not present any visible signs to the unaided eye. Many people insist on standing up after a fall, only to collapse when they put weight on a fractured hip or leg, which can cause further injury.

## Witnessed and assisted falls

### Breaking a fall

If a nurse is assisting a patient and notices the patient is about to fall, the nurse should pull the patient toward him or her, supporting the patient under the arms. The nurse should then bring his or her outside leg back a step for support and gently slide the patient down the angled front leg. After checking to ensure that the patient sustained no immediate, serious injuries, the nurse should follow hospital procedures for checking vital signs, getting help, and returning the patient to bed.

### Assessment

Patient assessment is easier if the fall was witnessed, because the cause of the fall may be known, and whoever witnessed the fall will know whether the individual hit his or her head. However, even if the fall was witnessed, the patient must be fully evaluated for injury.

## Unwitnessed falls

If a staff member reaches a patient after a fall has occurred, he or she must quickly assess the patient. While conducting a post-fall assessment, consider the following:

- Assess the patient—what is wrong, and what is the most severe problem?
  - Is he or she conscious? Breathing? Does he or she have a pulse?
  - Has a life-threatening injury occurred? Are there signs of shock?
  - Are there visible signs of injury, such as bleeding?
  - Can the patient tell you what happened?

- Assess the situation—what caused the problem?

- Remove the patient from imminent danger, if necessary.

- Provide and maintain comfort and keep the patient immobile.

- Check for responsiveness, and ask the patient what happened.

- Check vital signs.

- Check for injuries such as:
  - Scrapes or abrasions
  - Bumps, swelling, or bruises
  - Skin cuts or lacerations
  - Sprains or broken bones
  - Obvious bumps or bleeding from the head
- Ask about pain and note verbal complaints or facial grimacing.

- Look for asymmetry of extremities or limbs of different sizes.

- Check range of motion of extremities.

- Watch for anything unusual in appearance or behavior.

# First aid

After performing initial assessment on patients who have fallen, you should administer first aid. Take the following steps:

- Respond—call for help. Depending on the situation, call your supervisor or the patient's physician.

- Remove any danger to others or yourself.

- Perform CPR, if necessary.

- Apply pressure to stop bleeding, if necessary.

- Keep the patient warm and elevate his or her feet.

- Make the patient comfortable.

- If you must move the patient because he or she is in a life-threatening position, carefully support the neck and spine. Stop moving at the first sign of increased pain.

- Provide reassurance and support to the patient and keep him or her warm and safe.

- Prevent further embarrassment by making sure the patient is covered and modesty is preserved. If you have help, have someone stay with the patient while someone else moves curious onlookers out of the way. Onlookers may also need reassurance.

- Communicate. Inform the people who need to know about the fall and document the incident in your hospital records and in an incident report, according to hospital policy.

The first responder at the scene of a fall is the person who is best prepared to document both in the medical record and complete the incident report. Completing an incident report does not eliminate the need to document the fall within the medical record.

# Monitoring after the fall

As a general rule, a physician should examine any indication of injury as soon as possible. A physician should immediately evaluate any head trauma. Other injuries, such as suspected or obvious fractures, also require rapid treatment, as do symptoms of cardiac or neurological crisis.

Nurses must be especially alert to possible injuries for several days after a fall. Delayed discovery of a hip or other fracture is a common occurrence. Watch for the following indications that anything is different about the patient:

- Altered gait or limp
- Unusual hesitation or slowness when moving
- Verbal complaints of pain
- Nonverbal indications of pain, such as facial grimaces
- Loss of appetite
- Serious bruising of any part of the body
- Redness or warmth to any part of the body
- Favoring of an appendage, such as not using an arm or hand

Never assume that a patient's complaint of pain or signs of injury are simply the minor effects of taking a tumble and don't indicate anything serious. Just because a doctor evaluates someone and declares him or her uninjured does not rule out an undetected insult to some part of the body, with symptoms that may surface later. Every continuing complaint of unresolved pain must be investigated thoroughly. Every new symptom or change of condition requires careful examination. The consequences of not following these guidelines can be severe, such as permanent crippling injuries or even death.

A patient's plan of care following any fall should include additional checks or monitoring of the patient's status for several days. The frequency of those checks depends on the individual patient and the circumstances, but in many cases, once or twice a shift is sufficient for three or four days. Document these extra monitoring efforts or assessments and the results, even if no additional symptoms arise. It shows diligence and conscientious care when there is a clear effort to follow up after a fall.

| FIGURE 6.1 | Head-injury monitoring plan |
|---|---|

1. Use the head-injury monitoring plan form to document observations.

2. Check on the patient at least once every two to three hours for a minimum of 24 hours, and at least once per shift after that until 72 hours (three full days) have passed or as the physician orders.

3. At every check, look for signs of brain injury following the 12 signs listed on the monitoring plan.

4. If there is no evidence of a particular symptom, check "none" in the box by that symptom. Do this for all 12 symptoms.

5. Take the patient's respirations and blood pressure at every check time and write them on the form.

6. If any of the 12 signs are noticed, if the patient's pulse or blood pressure are unusually low, or if anything else seems unusual, follow appropriate setting response. In an inpatient setting, increase monitoring, consult attending physician, and implement code/emergency response procedures as appropriate. In an outpatient setting/nursing home, increase monitoring, consult attending physician, implement code/emergency response procedures as appropriate, and call 911 if necessary.

7. Notify the administrator, doctor, and family of the situation.

**FIGURE 6.1** — Head-injury monitoring plan (cont.)

Instructions: Use this plan whenever a patient hits his or her head or as instructed by physician. Begin monitoring immediately after injury. Check the patient for these signs of serious injury as often as instructed, but no less often than once every shift, for at least 72 hours after the injury occurred. Document the use of this plan on the communication log. When completed, file this plan with the patient service notes.

If any of these signs are observed, follow appropriate setting response.

| Write date, time, and signature. For each box below, check "none" or follow appropriate setting response if signs are observed. | Date: | | | | | | | |
|---|---|---|---|---|---|---|---|---|
| | Time: | | | | | | | |
| | Sign: | | | | | | | |
| 1. Loss of consciousness, unusual drowsiness, difficulty waking | ☐ None / If present, follow appropriate setting response | ☐ None / If present, follow appropriate setting response | ☐ None / If present, follow appropriate setting response | ☐ None / If present, follow appropriate setting response | ☐ None / If present, follow appropriate setting response | ☐ None / If present, follow appropriate setting response | ☐ None / If present, follow appropriate setting response | ☐ None / If present, follow appropriate setting response |
| 2. Headache or head pain that doesn't get better within four hours of head injury; stiff neck | ☐ None / If present, follow appropriate setting response | ☐ None / If present, follow appropriate setting response | ☐ None / If present, follow appropriate setting response | ☐ None / If present, follow appropriate setting response | ☐ None / If present, follow appropriate setting response | ☐ None / If present, follow appropriate setting response | ☐ None / If present, follow appropriate setting response | ☐ None / If present, follow appropriate setting response |
| 3. Blurred or double vision; loss of or change in vision | ☐ None / Yes? Follow appropriate setting response | ☐ None / Yes? Follow appropriate setting response | ☐ None / Yes? Follow appropriate setting response | ☐ None / Yes? Follow appropriate setting response | ☐ None / Yes? Follow appropriate setting response | ☐ None / Yes? Follow appropriate setting response | ☐ None / Yes? Follow appropriate setting response | ☐ None / Yes? Follow appropriate setting response |
| 4. Slowed or slurred speech; difficulty speaking | ☐ None / Yes? Follow appropriate setting response | ☐ None / Yes? Follow appropriate setting response | ☐ None / Yes? Follow appropriate setting response | ☐ None / Yes? Follow appropriate setting response | ☐ None / Yes? Follow appropriate setting response | ☐ None / Yes? Follow appropriate setting response | ☐ None / Yes? Follow appropriate setting response | ☐ None / Yes? Follow appropriate setting response |
| 5. Dizziness, poor coordination, dropping things, feeling faint, staggering, weakness, tingling, numbness, falling | ☐ None / If symptoms present, follow appropriate setting response | ☐ None / If symptoms present, follow appropriate setting response | ☐ None / If symptoms present, follow appropriate setting response | ☐ None / If symptoms present, follow appropriate setting response | ☐ None / If symptoms present, follow appropriate setting response | ☐ None / If symptoms present, follow appropriate setting response | ☐ None / If symptoms present, follow appropriate setting response | ☐ None / If symptoms present, follow appropriate setting response |
| 6. Abnormal behavior, irritability, confusion, restlessness, poor concentration, sadness, memory loss, personality change | ☐ None / If symptoms present, follow appropriate setting response | ☐ None / If symptoms present, follow appropriate setting response | ☐ None / If symptoms present, follow appropriate setting response | ☐ None / If symptoms present, follow appropriate setting response | ☐ None / If symptoms present, follow appropriate setting response | ☐ None / If symptoms present, follow appropriate setting response | ☐ None / If symptoms present, follow appropriate setting response | ☐ None / If symptoms present, follow appropriate setting response |
| 7. Decreased breathing rate (below 10 or as instructed), low blood pressure (below 90/50 or as instructed). **Write R & BP here.** | Resp: BP: / If either are low, follow appropriate setting response | Resp: BP: / If either are low, follow appropriate setting response | Resp: BP: / If either are low, follow appropriate setting response | Resp: BP: / If either are low, follow appropriate setting response | Resp: BP: / If either are low, follow appropriate setting response | Resp: BP: / If either are low, follow appropriate setting response | Resp: BP: / If either are low, follow appropriate setting response | Resp: BP: / If either are low, follow appropriate setting response |
| 8. Bleeding or fluid drainage from ears, nose, or head | ☐ None / Yes? Follow appropriate setting response | ☐ None / Yes? Follow appropriate setting response | ☐ None / Yes? Follow appropriate setting response | ☐ None / Yes? Follow appropriate setting response | ☐ None / Yes? Follow appropriate setting response | ☐ None / Yes? Follow appropriate setting response | ☐ None / Yes? Follow appropriate setting response | ☐ None / Yes? Follow appropriate setting response |
| 9. Nausea or vomiting | ☐ None / Yes? Follow appropriate setting response | ☐ None / Yes? Follow appropriate setting response | ☐ None / Yes? Follow appropriate setting response | ☐ None / Yes? Follow appropriate setting response | ☐ None / Yes? Follow appropriate setting response | ☐ None / Yes? Follow appropriate setting response | ☐ None / Yes? Follow appropriate setting response | ☐ None / Yes? Follow appropriate setting response |
| 10. Swelling or indentation at site of injury | ☐ None / Yes? Follow appropriate setting response | ☐ None / Yes? Follow appropriate setting response | ☐ None / Yes? Follow appropriate setting response | ☐ None / Yes? Follow appropriate setting response | ☐ None / Yes? Follow appropriate setting response | ☐ None / Yes? Follow appropriate setting response | ☐ None / Yes? Follow appropriate setting response | ☐ None / Yes? Follow appropriate setting response |
| 11. Uncontrolled shaking or trembling | ☐ None / Yes? Follow appropriate setting response | ☐ None / Yes? Follow appropriate setting response | ☐ None / Yes? Follow appropriate setting response | ☐ None / Yes? Follow appropriate setting response | ☐ None / Yes? Follow appropriate setting response | ☐ None / Yes? Follow appropriate setting response | ☐ None / Yes? Follow appropriate setting response | ☐ None / Yes? Follow appropriate setting response |
| 12. Eyes: One pupil not the same size as the other | ☐ None / Yes? Follow appropriate setting response | ☐ None / Yes? Follow appropriate setting response | ☐ None / Yes? Follow appropriate setting response | ☐ None / Yes? Follow appropriate setting response | ☐ None / Yes? Follow appropriate setting response | ☐ None / Yes? Follow appropriate setting response | ☐ None / Yes? Follow appropriate setting response | ☐ None / Yes? Follow appropriate setting response |

**Evidence-Based Falls Prevention, Second Edition**

# Head injuries

A patient who sustains a blow to the head should first be examined by a physician, who will then provide orders for specific monitoring. Even in the event of normal test results, x-rays, and a physician's certification that the patient does not have a serious injury, careful monitoring is still indicated for at least 72 hours after the fall. It is not uncommon for a brain injury to present itself days later. If the patient is not closely watched and the problems are not identified as early as possible, significant additional damage can be incurred.

You may not know whether a patient hit his or her head, particularly if the patient has a poor memory or is cognitively impaired. When you know or even suspect that a patient has sustained a head injury as a result of a fall, follow the procedures outlined in Figure 6.1.

# Documentation

Recording specific information about every fall is an essential component of fall response and prevention. There are a number of reasons that careful documentation is required:

- To plan effective interventions, the care team must have good information about past falls, including their causes and outcomes. Preventing patient falls requires accurate historical data as well as current assessment information.

- Regulatory bodies look closely at falls, and thorough documentation may be the only evidence of appropriate response and follow-up. State surveyors want to see the complete story when they read a patient's record, including assessment, response, interventions, and outcomes. Inadequate documentation often produces citations for the hospital.

- Sometimes a fall prompts legal action in the form of a civil suit or even criminal neglect charges. In the eyes of the law, care that isn't documented wasn't done. Thorough documentation protects the institution and its employees.

- Quality improvement must be based on data that can only come from careful documentation and tracking of falls, interventions, and outcomes.

| FIGURE 6.2 | Initial note documentation |
| --- | --- |

- Date/time of the fall.

- Report of the fall:

  - What happened?
  - Any identifiable causes?
  - How was the patient discovered?
  - Was the fall witnessed or unwitnessed?
  - Did an injury occur?
  - Who else was involved, if anyone?
  - What did the patient say about the fall?

- Nature of the injury, if any:

  - Location of injury
  - Size of injury
  - Open areas/bleeding/fractures
  - Reported pain
  - Suspected or actual head trauma

- Time of fall/injury.

- Did the patient require surgery?

- Who was notified, how were they notified, and at what time were they notified?

- What were the physician's orders?

- Was report of current status called to the emergency department?

- Was there any report from the emergency department later?

- Was the patient transferred to another hospital? Where? For what?

Useful documentation requires more than a simple recording of the event in the service notes. Keep at least three distinct information records about every fall: the service or nursing note narrative, the incident report, and the incident-tracking record. In addition, the service plan or care plan should reflect appropriate interventions in response to a fall, including an incident report.

Figure 6.2 lists all of the documentation to include in the initial incident report. This information will be used to track falls and outcomes in the hospital, giving risk and quality managers the data they need to identify problem areas and implement changes. Depending on local regulations, incident reports are sometimes protected from discovery in the event of legal action, which makes them a good place to note details about risk and quality issues that might not belong in the service record. Regardless of whether they are protected, the incident report should be a vehicle for noting the specifics of cause and effect, employee action and patient response, notifications to supervisors, and outcomes. If a fall prompts legal or regulatory action, the incident report can demonstrate the correct response of the employee or hospital and fill in gaps often left in narrative notes.

## Recommended nurse documentation for falls

Complete documentation as soon after the fall as possible. This documentation is part of the patient's permanent record and is best written while the event, your assessment, any interventions, the patient's responses, and the outcomes are fresh in your mind. Figure 6.3 examines what information to include in a nurse's documentation of a fall.

Different hospitals find different tools useful in supporting their chosen policies and procedures, and it is rare that one particular tool will work well for everyone.

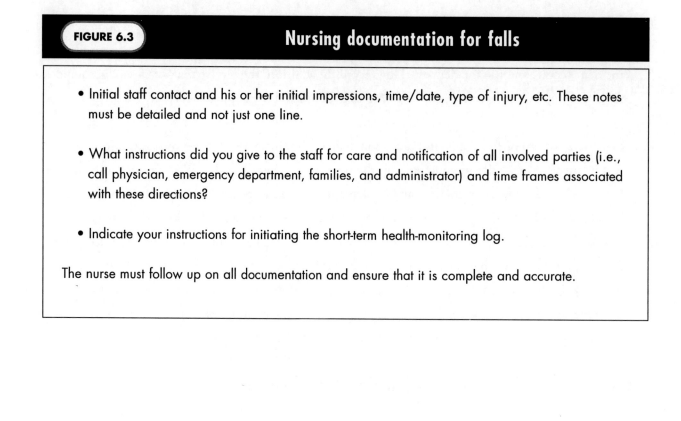

**FIGURE 6.3**      Nursing documentation for falls

- Initial staff contact and his or her initial impressions, time/date, type of injury, etc. These notes must be detailed and not just one line.

- What instructions did you give to the staff for care and notification of all involved parties (i.e., call physician, emergency department, families, and administrator) and time frames associated with these directions?

- Indicate your instructions for initiating the short-term health-monitoring log.

The nurse must follow up on all documentation and ensure that it is complete and accurate.

# CHAPTER 7:

## Pediatric falls

# Pediatric falls

## Learning objectives

After reading this chapter, the participant should be able to:

- Identify four categories of pediatric falls

## Childhood falls: The healthcare perspective

In the world of fall prevention, pediatric falls has become a major initiative. As the most common cause of injury visits to the emergency department for young children[1], falls account for an estimated 2.5 million emergency visits annually.[2] Falls are also the leading cause of nonfatal injuries to children up to 14 years of age.

### National Patient Safety Goals

From a hospital's perspective, children are largely unpredictable, but that does not mean that fall risk prevention programs do not apply to pediatrics. In its FAQs for the 2007 National Patient Safety Goals, The Joint Commission clarified that children are not exempt from the fall risk National Patient Safety Goal. It stated that healthcare facilities need to develop criteria to identify and screen populations of children at risk for falls, and that those at-risk children need to be assessed and protected.[3]

> **According to The Joint Commission:**
>
> 1. "Dropped" patients (e.g., infants) are outside the scope of this safety goal
>
> 2. There should not be a blanket exemption for pediatrics
>
> 3. Criteria should be developed to assist in identifying populations of children who are at risk of being harmed from falls
>
> 4. All children should be "screened" to determine whether they are in an "at-risk" population
>
> 5. Any child who is in an "at-risk" population should be assessed and protected
>
> *Source: The Joint Commission, FAQs for the 2007 National Patient Safety Goals*

## Identifying children at risk

Many hospitalized children are at risk of falling, and children's hospitals have long provided a high nurse-to-patient ratio to help supervise and protect children from injury. Only recently has there been research to predict whether specific populations or characteristics put certain children at a higher risk than others.

Research has shown that certain medicines have been noted to increase pediatric falls risk. Seizure medication was noted as a risk factor in a recent study, and antihistamines have been shown to cause sedation or drowsiness and, therefore, may increase the child's fall risk. Additionally, a child who has received an orthopedic diagnosis was concluded to be at a higher risk of falling.[4]

Nurses should note any changes in the child's mental status, such as confusion after an operation or episodes of disorientation (or, for infants, any lack of response to auditory, tactile, or visual stimuli). Additionally, any history of falls for the child should be noted, if the fall was not developmental (e.g., the child learning to walk).

Children under the age of 36 months need a watchful eye, particularly those who are under one year of age. Children who are mobility impaired can also be at a higher risk of falling; such children can be identified by their need to use furniture or walls when they walk, or their need for crutches, a walker, or another assistive tool.

Several predictor models are currently being tested to help identify children at risk of falling. The Children's Hospital at Saint Francis, located in Tulsa, OK, for example, has developed the following tool (called CHAMPS, as seen in Figure 7.1) to help identify risk factors for pediatric falls and actions to be taken.[5]

## Categorizing pediatric falls

It can be difficult to determine the actions a hospitalized child may take, and the hospital staff must serve in a parent-surrogate role when parents are not present to help monitor their child's activities. However, there are measures that a hospital can take to minimize falls in the pediatric unit.

Pediatric falls should be categorized by type of fall, rather than merely counting the number of falls that take place. Classifying falls provides direction for how to best intervene to prevent further falls. Several types of falls can be witnessed among hospitalized children:[6]

- **Developmental falls:** These falls are "normal" and refer to tumbles that take place while a child is learning to stand, walk, run, or pivot. Often, children under age three will experience developmental falls as they learn to balance. Development falls are normal and should not be prevented as that can delay the child's learning. The focus with developmental falls is the elimination of any injury by making the hospital environment as safe as or safer than the child's home environment.

- **Accidental falls:** These falls are due to misjudgment on the part of the patient, family member, nurse, or other involved person. This includes leaving side rails down on a bed, tripping over an object that was left in the way (such as an IV pole or electrical cord), or having poor lighting or slippery floors. Accidental falls can be prevented through environmental surveillance rounds and educational support to families and staff members.

- **Anticipated physical/physiological falls:** These falls occur as a result of characteristics that are intrinsic to a patient or population. Characteristics found to be predictive of hospital falls in children may include orthopedic, muscular/skeletal conditions, seizures or the need for use of antiepileptic medications, the need for physical or occupational therapy assistance, or certain psychiatric disorders (ADHD, oppositional defiance disorders, or compulsive/combative disorders).

| FIGURE 7.1 | CHAMPS pediatric fall risk assessment tool |
|---|---|

The first four items are risk factors and the second two are nursing interventions.

| Risk Factor | Yes | No | Comments |
|---|---|---|---|
| Change in mental status | | | Episodes of disorientation, dizziness, confusion related to postop status, medication (high dose of narcotics, rapid weaning of sedation), or illness. Newborn/infant indicators may include irritability; agitation; inconsolability; nonresponsiveness to auditory, visual, or tactile stimuli. |
| History of falls | | | Accidental fall = a developmentally inappropriate fall. Patient has experienced an accidental fall recently. |
| Age less than 36 months | | | Answer yes - if less than 36 months of age chronologically or developmentally. |
| Mobility impairment | | | Mobility includes ability to get in/out of bed/crib unassisted as well as ability to utilize bathroom without assistance. Yes – patient needs help of furniture/walls to ambulate. Yes – patient needs crutches, walker, or other assistive device to ambulate. Yes – patient needs assistance of one or two people to ambulate. Yes – patient is less than one year of age. |

© 2007 HCPro, Inc.     **Evidence-Based Falls Prevention, Second Edition**

| FIGURE 7.1 | CHAMPS pediatric fall risk assessment tool (cont.) | | |
| --- | --- | --- | --- |

| Risk Factor | Yes | No | Comments |
| --- | --- | --- | --- |
| Parental involvement | | | • Partners in prevention, parent education.<br>• Over 80% of children's falls in a hospital occur when a caregiver is in attendance. Falls are more likely to occur with getting out of bed or going to the bathroom.<br>• Use the call light for bathroom and/or assistance getting out of bed. |
| Safety | | | Implementation of interventions:<br>• Reeducate on asking for assistance in getting out of bed<br>• Reeducate to maintain crib rails up at all times if child is unsupervised<br>• Reassess use of siderails<br>• Night light in room<br>• Consider change of bed to crib/other bed type as developmentally appropriate<br>• Offer child life consults as appropriate to provide diversion activity<br>• Call light within reach of caregiver/patient<br>• Appropriate use of side-rails/crib rails for prevention of falls<br>• Room free of clutter<br>• Assess whether need to move closer to nursing station for unattended/high-risk fall |

*Source: Razmus, I., and Wilson, D. Reprinted with permission.*

- **Unanticipated physical/physiological falls:** These falls take place due to a child's unpredicted response to a medical regimen. The child may have been admitted for another reason but might become dehydrated and faint as a result of a side effect of a medication or an unknown health condition. This type of fall often cannot be predicted, but future falls can be prevented with the implementation of an appropriate fall prevention plan of care.

## A step toward prevention

Nursing staff can take important steps toward keeping young patients safe:

- **Partner with parents.** More than 80% of pediatric falls occur when parents are present.[7] Thus, it is vital to educate parents on how to keep their child protected from fall-related injuries. Remind parents not to bring side rails down, for example, and to keep curtains open so that nurses can see the child.

- **Keep the environment safe.** Make sure the room and hallways surrounding the child are kept orderly and that furniture and equipment are not in the child's path:
  - Check that sharp corners are padded
  - Make sure there is adequate lighting (leave a night light on, etc.)
  - Keep all floors dry
  - Remove furniture near windows that children can climb on
  - Store personal items within reach
  - Make nonskid footwear available
  - Verify that bed wheels are locked and brakes are on

- **Mark the territory.** By putting colorful stickers by a patient's name at the nurses' station or placing a "Caution" sign on a patient's door, you can alert others that the child is at high risk of falling. Caregivers will then know to take proper measures to ensure the child's safety. Hospitals can provide annual education to staff members regarding age and developmental characteristics to take into consideration when caring for children of various ages.

- **Stay by the child's side.** Accompany the child as he or she walks to the bathroom or if the child is walking with medical equipment, such as crutches or a cast. Encourage the use of grab bars in the bathroom. Also, take the time to assist the child as he or she gets out of bed for the first time. Monitor children closely the first few nights that they are hospitalized as they get used to this new environment to ensure that they do not fall out of bed or wander.

- **Encourage family-centered care.** Encourage parents to participate in the care and monitoring of their child. Provide a place for parents to stay with their child at night. Remember to assess how attentive parents are to their child's needs and behavior and intervene if parents are unable to set safe and appropriate behavior limits for their child.

## *Adolescents*

When compared with much younger children, older children or teenagers might be harder to entertain, especially as they begin to get better. As boredom ensues, the adolescent might want to get up and walk around, and will hesitate to ask for assistance (such as before heading to the bathroom).

Nurses should be aware that an adolescent is often unwilling to ask for help, and that it is thus important to increase patient surveillance. The young patient should be reminded that he or she is not bothering or disturbing the nurse by asking for assistance. Make sure the patient knows that you have the time and that he or she should not feel burdensome or embarrassed to ask for help.

# References

1. University of Maryland Medical Center (UMMC), Baltimore 2007.

2. Fox, M. E. *www.foxinjurylaw.com/CM/Custom/Personal-Injury-ENews.asp*. Visited 8/14/07.

3. The Joint Commission (2007). "FAQs for the 2007 National Patient Safety Goals." *www.joint-commission.org*. Visited 8/15/07).

4. Graf, Elaine, PhD, RN, PNP, research and funding coordinator for Children's Memorial Medical Center, Chicago. Presentation, November 2005: "Pediatric Hospital Falls: Development of a Predictor Model to Guide Pediatric Clinical Practice."

5. Newman, E., Razmus, I., Smith, R., and Wilson, D. (2006). "Falls in hospitalized children." *Pediatric Nursing* 32(6): 568–572.

6. Graf, Elaine, PhD, RN, PNP, research and funding coordinator for Children's Memorial Medical Center, Chicago.

7. The Children's Hospital at Saint Francis, Saint Francis Health System, 2004.

# Nursing education instructional guide

**Evidence-Based
Falls Prevention:
A Study Guide for Nurses,
Second Edition**

# Nursing education instructional guide Evidence-Based Falls Prevention: A Study Guide for Nurses, Second Edition

## Target audience:

Directors of nursing

VPs of patient services

Chief nursing officers

Staff development coordinators

Quality directors

Directors of patient safety

Risk managers

## Statement of need:

This book provides an educational study guide for nurses to assist them in delivering safe, effective care. The guide explains how to protect your patients from errors and harm associated with one of the newest National Patient Safety Goals—preventing patient falls. Patient falls have been reported in acute care for some time but only now have reached the level of a formal and measurable national goal through The Joint Commission (formerly JCAHO). The guide will help fulfill the Joint Commission requirement to educate nurses on patient safety, specifically about the National Patient Safety Goal on patient falls.

# Educational objectives:

Upon completion of this activity, participants should be able to:

- State a goal for performing an assessment
- Explain why documentation is important
- Describe the two phases of nursing assessment
- Identify elements of the functional screen
- Define a fall
- Identify several nonmodifiable intrinsic fall risk factors
- List examples of modifiable risk factors
- List functional risk factor modifications
- Describe recommendations for preventing falls in the cognitively impaired
- List specific medical conditions responsible for falls that are often overlooked
- Identify hospitalwide steps that may reduce the risk of falls
- List modifiable risk factors that a good falls-prevention program should address
- Identify the three main elements of a falls-prevention program
- Identify elements that should be included in a multifactorial intervention program
- Formulate questions to ask after a fall takes place in order to respond appropriately
- Describe factors to consider when conducting a post-fall assessment of an unwitnessed fall
- Identify three distinct information records that must be maintained for every fall
- Identify four categories of pediatric falls

## *Faculty*

Carole Eldridge, DNP, RN, CNAA-BC—Carole Eldridge was the primary author of
this publication.

Elaine Graf, PhD, RN, PNP—Elaine Graf reviewed the content of this publication.

## *Accreditation/designation statement*

This educational activity for two contact hours is provided by HCPro, Inc., HCPro, Inc. is accredited as a provider of continuing nursing education by the American Nurses Credentialing Center's Commission on Accreditation.

### *Disclosure statements*

Carole Eldridge and Elaine Graf have declared that they have no commercial/financial vested interest in this activity.

# Instructions

In order to be eligible to receive your nursing contact hour(s) for this activity, you are required to do the following:

1. Read the book
2. Complete the exam
3. Complete the evaluation
4. Provide your contact information in the space provided on the exam and evaluation
5. Submit the exam and evaluation to HCPro, Inc.

Please provide all of the information requested above and mail or fax your completed exam, program evaluation, and contact information to:

HCPro, Inc.
ATTN: Continuing Education Department
200 Hoods Lane
Marblehead, MA 01945
Tel: 877/727-1728
Fax: 781/639/2982

# Nursing education exam

Name:

_____

Title:

_____

Facility name:

_____

Address:

_____

Address:

_____

City: _____  State: _____ ZIP: _____

Phone number: _____  Fax number: _____

E-mail:

_____

Nursing license number:

_____

(ANCC requires a unique identifier for each learner)

1.  **What is the goal of performing an assessment and developing a plan of care?**
    a. Improve outcomes for the patient
    b. Determine cost-efficient methods of treatment
    c. Delegate tasks to staff nurses
    d. Identify responsibilities of staff

2.  **Objective data is:**
    a. Obtained from the patient directly
    b. Observable
    c. Difficult to obtain
    d. Measurable

3. Documentation:

   a. Fails to demonstrate compliance with the standards for assessment and care of patients

   b. Shows that the patient's condition was not thoroughly assessed

   c. Is not the responsibility of the nurse

   d. Proves that the patient's status was continually evaluated

4. **What are the two phases of nursing assessment?**

   a.  Problem identification and observation

   b. Data collection and problem identification

   c. Data collection and interview

   d. Observation and data collection

5. **The functional screen contains which of the following elements?**

   a. A lack of risk indicators

   b. Patient allergies

   c. Patient's food preferences

   d. How many, or to what degree, indicators must be present

6. **All patients must have an assessment completed by a registered nurse (RN) within _____ of admission, to determine the patient's need for nursing care.**

   a. 1 hour

   b. 12 hours

   c. 24 hours

   d. 48 hours

7. **A fall is:**

   a. Unpreventable

   b. Any sudden, unintentional change in position that causes an individual to land at a lower level, on an object, on the floor, or on the ground

   c. When a patient slightly trips but remains upright

   d. Only caused by environmental hazards

8. All of the following traits are nonmodifiable fall risk factors except:

    a. Age

    b. Race

    c. Nutrition

    d. Gender

9. Which of the following is not a modifiable risk factor?

    a. Inactivity

    b. Inadequate nutrition

    c. Excessive alcohol intake

    d. Poor balance

10. Approximately _____ of falls result primarily from extrinsic factors in the environment.

    a. 25%

    b. 75%

    c. 50%

    d. 10%

11. Patients with combined gait and balance difficulties are _____ more likely to fall than those with normal gait and balance.

    a. two times

    b. four times

    c. three times

    d. not

12. The inner ear perceives _____, helping to make the necessary accommodations to adjust posture and exert muscular control.

    a. gravity

    b. sound

    c. depth

    d. light

 **Evidence-Based Falls Prevention, Second Edition**

13.  Medical conditions that increase fall risk include all of the following except:

a. Vascular disorders

b. Neuromuscular disorders

c. Musculoskeletal disorders

d. Eating disorders

14. Which of the following is a functional risk factor modification?

a. Nutrition

b. Gender

c. Race

d. Age

15. What is one recommendation for preventing falls in the cognitively impaired?

a. Assume a patient can't comply with a modification because he or she is cognitively impaired

b. Consider a broad range of fall causes

c. Have the cognitively impaired patient wear socks and shoes so he or she can feel the floor

d. Do not attempt to determine the direction in which a patient will fall because patients with degenerative dementia develop unpredictable falling patterns

16. What is a medical condition responsible for falls that is often overlooked?

a. Diabetes

b. Stomach flu

c. Obesity

d. Orthostatic hypotension (OH)

17.  What are two results of cognitive impairment?

a. Loss of judgment and appetite

b. Loss of visual acuity and hearing

c. Loss of visual acuity and judgment

d. Loss of hearing and judgment

18. In a fall-prevention program, a patient's medication regimen should be audited to flag anyone taking more than _____ medications routinely.

    a. three

    b. four

    c. two

    d. five

19. What steps can hospitals take to reduce the overall risk of falls?

    a. Only review certain patient medication

    b. Implement a system in which nurses are encouraged to identify who is to blame for a fall

    c. Keep patients out of the loop so that nurses can better focus

    d. Educate staff using programs to raise awareness of fall risk and teach prevention measures

20. A good fall-prevention program addresses all of the following modifiable risk factors except:

    a. Sedatives

    b. Orthostatic hypotension (OH)

    c. Use of more than two medications

    d. Foot problems

21. What is one main element of a fall-prevention program?

    a. Disallowing patient input during program development

    b. Keeping other involved healthcare workers in the dark concerning risk factors

    c. Modifying the risk factors without family involvement

    d. Assessing the patients to identify the risk factors facing each individual and the hospital as a whole

22. What element should not be included in a multifactorial intervention program?

    a. Gait training

    b. Modification of medication regimens

    c. Treatment of postural hypotension

    d. Lack of patient input

     **Evidence-Based Falls Prevention, Second Edition**

**23. Root cause is:**

a. A method for ascertaining blame after an incident

b. The underlying reason that something occurred

c. Not the committee's responsibility

d. The only reason something happened; there are never several root causes of an incident

**24. What question should you ask to determine the root cause of a fall?**

a. Was the cause intrinsic or extrinsic?

b. Whose fault was the fall?

c. How much will the fall cost the hospital in necessary repairs of environmental hazards?

d. Who was on duty when the fall occurred?

**25. What two questions should you ask after a fall to determine the appropriate response?**

a. Why did the patient fall? What injuries have occurred?

b. Who is at fault? Why did the patient fall?

c. How many times has the patient fallen before? What injuries have occurred?

d. Where was the patient when the fall occurred? Who is at fault?

**26. What is one factor to consider when conducting a post-fall assessment in an unwitnessed fall?**

a. Name of patient

b. Time of the fall

c. Date of fall

d. Cause of the problem

**27. What three distinct information records should you keep about every fall?**

a. Service or nursing note narrative, questions asked of the patient at the time of the fall, notes about whose oversight caused the fall

b. Service or nursing note narrative, incident report, incident-tracking record

c. Service or nursing note narrative, notes about whose oversight caused fall, incident report

d. Incident report, incident-tracking record, summary of comorbid conditions of patient

28. What information should be included in a nurse's documentation of a fall?

    a. One-line notes about the type of injury

    b. Instructions given to staff about notification of all involved parties

    c. Weight of the patient

    d. Written summary of who he/she believes is to blame for the fall

29. All of the following information should be included in an initial incident report except:

    a. Date/time of the fall

    b. Nature of the injury

    c. Physician orders

    d. Height of the patient

30. What is an indication of a possible injury after the fall?

    a. Increase in appetite

    b. Favoring of an appendage, such as not using an arm or a leg

    c. Unusual quickness when moving

    d. Coolness to any part of the body

31. Which of the following is not a category of pediatric falls?

    a. Anticipated falls

    b. Accidental falls

    c. Developmental falls

    d. Consistent falls

# Nursing education evaluation

Name:

_____

Title:

_____

Facility name:

_____

Address:

_____

Address: _____

City: _____ State: _____ ZIP: _____

Phone number: _____ Fax number: _____

E-mail: _____

Nursing license number: _____

(ANCC requires a unique identifier for each learner)

**1. This activity met the following learning objectives:**

a.) Stated the goal of performing an assessment and developing a plan of care

Strongly disagree    1        2        3        4        5        Strongly agree

b.) Described why documentation is important

Strongly disagree    1        2        3        4        5        Strongly agree

c.) Stated the two phases of nursing assessment

Strongly disagree    1        2        3        4        5        Strongly agree

d.) Defined a fall

Strongly disagree    1        2        3        4        5        Strongly agree

e.) Identified several nonmodifiable intrinsic fall risk factors

Strongly disagree    1        2        3        4        5        Strongly agree

f.) Listed examples of modifiable risk factors

Strongly disagree    1        2        3        4        5        Strongly agree

g.) Listed functional risk factor modifications

Strongly disagree    1        2        3        4        5        Strongly agree

h.) Identified recommendations for preventing falls in the cognitively impaired

Strongly disagree    1        2        3        4        5        Strongly agree

i.) Listed specific medical conditions responsible for falls that are often overlooked

Strongly disagree    1      2      3      4      5      Strongly agree

j.) Identified hospitalwide steps that may reduce the risk of falls

Strongly disagree    1      2      3      4      5      Strongly agree

k.) Listed modifiable risk factors that a good fall-prevention program should address

Strongly disagree    1      2      3      4      5      Strongly agree

l.) Stated the three main elements of a fall-prevention program

Strongly disagree    1      2      3      4      5      Strongly agree

m.) Identified elements that should be included in a multifactorial intervention program

Strongly disagree    1      2      3      4      5      Strongly agree

n.) Listed questions to ask after a fall to determine the appropriate response

Strongly disagree    1      2      3      4      5      Strongly agree

o.) Stated factors to consider when conducting a postfall assessment in an unwitnessed fall

Strongly disagree    1      2      3      4      5      Strongly agree

p.) Identified three distinct information records you should keep about every fall

Strongly disagree    1      2      3      4      5      Strongly agree

**2. Objectives were related to the overall purpose/goal of the activity.**

Strongly disagree    1      2      3      4      5      Strongly agree

**3. This activity was related to my nursing activity needs.**

Strongly disagree    1      2      3      4      5      Strongly agree

**4. The exam for the activity was an accurate test of the knowledge gained.**

Strongly disagree    1      2      3      4      5      Strongly agree

**5. The activity avoided commercial bias or influence.**

Strongly disagree    1        2        3        4        5        Strongly agree

**6. This activity met my expectations.**

Strongly disagree    1        2        3        4        5        Strongly agree

**7. Will this learning activity enhance your professional nursing practice?**

Yes        No

**8. This educational method was an appropriate delivery tool for the nursing/clinical audience.**

Strongly disagree    1        2        3        4        5        Strongly agree

**9. How committed are you to making the behavioral changes suggested in this activity?**

a. Very committed

b. Somewhat committed

c. Not committed

**10. Please provide us with your degree.**

a. ADN

b. BSN

c. MSN

d. Other, please state

**11. Please provide us with your credentials.**

a. LVN                              d. NP

b. LPN                              e. Other, please state

c. RN

**12. Providing nursing contact hours for this product influenced my decision to buy it.**

Strongly disagree    1        2        3        4        5        Strongly agree

**13. I found the process to obtain my continuing education credits for this activity easy to complete.**

Strongly disagree    1        2        3        4        5        Strongly agree

14. If you did not find the process easy to complete, which of the following areas did you find the most difficult?

    a. Understanding the content of the activity

    b. Understanding the instructions

    c. Completing the exam

    d. Completing the evaluation

    e. Other, please state:

15. How much time did it take for you to complete this activity (this includes reading the book and completing the exam and the evaluation)? _____

16. If you have any comments on this activity, process, or selection of topics for nursing CE, please note them below.

_____

_____

_____

_____

17. Would you be interested in participating as a pilot tester for the development of future HCPro nursing education activities?

Yes   No

Thank you for completing this evaluation of our nursing CE activity!